HEALTH SOLUTIONS FOR
SLEEP

HEALTH SOLUTIONS FOR
SLEEP

A guide to easy sleep-promoting exercises,
sleep-friendly foods,
and more than 150 techniques clinically proven to rebalance
sleep-supportive body chemistry

DR. JAMES ROUSE

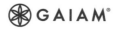

To my buddy, Dan. Sleep well, tiger.

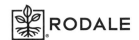

RODALE

WE **INSPIRE** AND **ENABLE** PEOPLE TO IMPROVE
THEIR LIVES AND THE WORLD AROUND THEM

Editor: Christine Bucks

Interior Book Designer: Joanna Williams

Cover Designer: Gaiam

Interior Photographers: Ron Derhacopian (poses); Mitch Mandel (food); Adam Brown (pages 12 and 38); and Gaiam (pages 22, 44, 90, 102, and 140)

Layout Designer: Donna Bellis

Copy Editor: Erana Bumbardatore

Product Specialist: Brenda Miller

Indexer: Nanette Bendyna

Rodale Organic Living Books

Executive Editor: Margot Schupf

Art Director: Patricia Field

Content Assembly Manager: Robert V. Anderson Jr.

Copy Manager: Nancy N. Bailey

We're always happy to hear from you. For questions or comments concerning the editorial content of this book, please write to:

Rodale Book Readers' Service

33 East Minor Street

Emmaus, PA 18098

Look for other Rodale books wherever books are sold. Or call us at (800) 848-4735.

For more information about Rodale magazines and books, visit us at

www.rodale.com

Library of Congress Cataloging-in-Publication Data

Rouse, James, date.
 Health solutions for sleep : a guide to easy sleep-promoting exercises, sleep-friendly foods, and more than 150 techniques clinically proven to rebalance sleep-supportive body chemistry / James Rouse.
  p.   cm.
 Includes index.
  ISBN 1–59250–150–8 paperback
  1. Insomnia—Popular works. I. Title.
RC548.R685 2003
616.8'498—dc21   2003010601

Distributed in the book trade by St. Martin's Press

2 4 6 8 10 9 7 5 3 1 paperback

Contents

Acknowledgments

I would like to acknowledge spirit and its guiding light and inner voice that has inspired me to follow my heart, act with compassion, love with zeal, and live with humility and gratitude for the gift of life.

This book represents a co-creative culmination of energies and expertise provided by colleagues, friends, family, and loved ones. Special thanks to my parents, Mom, Dad, Gail, and Bob, for establishing a foundation for me to build my dreams upon. To my sister and brother, Tamara and Bryan, I am grateful for your hearts and spirits, which you express with integrity and love. A heartfelt thank-you to all of my clients and patients who have continually inspired me through their commitment to healing and wholeness.

I am grateful for the experience, expertise, and encouraging enthusiasm of Kerry Eielson, whose energy and dedication to excellence allowed my thoughts to be represented so well in the pages of this book.

I am grateful for the opportunity to create with the gifted people at Rodale, Christine Bucks and Margot Schupf, and for having the benefit of their editorial expertise. I also wish to acknowledge fellow mind mapper Ron Derhacopian for your photographic excellence.

Thank you to Howard Ronder for your creative eyes and heart; to Andrea Lesky for your passionate persistence in bringing the workouts to life; and to Jirka Rysavy for sharing your courageous heart and vision with the whole world. To Lynn Powers, my friend and mentor, thank you for leading with your heart with passion, purpose, and impeccable grace.

Finally, I wish to acknowledge and dedicate this book to the greatest blessings and teachers of love in my life: my wife, Debra Jeanne, and my two most beautiful girls, Dakota and Elli. I appreciate your love, hugs, and laughter. You have given me the experience of having heaven on earth.

Your Body Knows Best

Sleep, just like breathing, should be one of the most natural things in the world. This seems especially true when you consider that it's something we spend a third of our lives doing. Yet most of us are not fulfilling this basic need. Sleep may be just something you know you need, or perhaps you even think of it as a nuisance. The only time you really think about sleep may be when you're not getting enough of it. Well, it's time to change that attitude. Sleep is fuel. It's restorative. It's a source of youthfulness, energy, focus, peace, and balance—and it's absolutely essential to living well.

You may have picked up this book because you want more sleep, but ask yourself this: Do you *value* sleep? How much effort are you willing to invest in rest? Think of your heart's deepest desire, your soul's greatest ambition. Would sleeping more rob you of that? On the other hand, could fatigue take it from you? Imagine if you slept great every night of your life and you felt radiant, energetic, balanced, and focused every morning. Can you imagine the probability of actualizing your potential?

Lack of sleep negatively impacts every part of your life, including your job performance, your mental and physical health, and your interactions with friends and family. It's time you started to assign a higher priority to getting consistent, quality rest. Begin by proactively assessing what you may have taken for granted. Your body has the instinctive ability to restore itself, every night, through a deep, deep sleep. Take advantage of this natural instinct.

FINDING YOUR UNIQUE SOLUTION TO SLEEP

Health Solutions for Sleep isn't about which sleeping pill is best for you. Rather, it's about basic principles including routine, mindfulness, movement, breath work, optimism, nutrition, and discovering and nurturing the things that bring you joy in life. In this book, I present you with a program you can tailor to rebuild your life in a way that augments your chemistry so you can get a good night's sleep every night. In time, difficulty sleeping will become a distant memory.

Sprinkled throughout the book you'll find boxes containing a "'To You' List." You can pick and choose suggestions from those lists that will help you change your lifestyle in small but vital ways—ways that will have a large impact on how well you sleep and on your life in general. By gradually implementing changes found in the "'To You' List," you'll feel happier, more peaceful, and full of vitality. And isn't that what you want?

A.M./P.M. Solutions

There's much more to sleeping deeply than whether you do or don't consume that cup of coffee or caffeinated soda in the afternoon. Insomnia is a 24-hour issue that requires around-the-clock care. From the moment you wake up, the food you eat, the way you move and breathe, the choices you make, and even your outlook all have a direct impact on your quality of sleep. That's why I've included daily improvements you can make to nutrition, breathing, exercise, and outlook— morning, noon, and night—for finding a long-term solution to difficulty sleeping. I also offer a variety of natural short-term sleep solutions that you can reach for when you're in the throes of a middle-of-the-night, wide-eyed-and-wired moment.

My goal is for you to find a permanent, natural solution (or combination of solutions) that treats your body as a whole. With this book, you will develop a multi-level support system that works to return your body to its natural rhythms.

As you read, compassionately work to discover what hinders or helps you rest. Pay attention to what's going on when you have trouble sleeping. Take a look at your daily routine, or lack thereof, and how food and exercise affect you. Also ask yourself, how much sleep do you personally need? How do you manipulate your body's chemistry with chemicals, routines, and habits that keep you going and going?

In asking these questions about your lifestyle, you'll reach a deeper understanding of the way your body works. During the process, you'll discover a clearer understanding of yourself and begin to move toward a truer, more defined picture of who you are and what you want out of life.

A Naturopathic Approach

You can't sustain good health without adequate sleep, a nutritionally rich diet, a positive mental attitude, and exercise. These are the basic tenets to high-level wellness. Optimum wellness is like a quilt, and sleep is one of the patches. This, a sustainable model of wellness, is the idea behind the naturopathic approach. It doesn't take years of imbalance to do the damage; you compromise your health every time you go four or five consecutive days and nights without healthy foods, conscious movement, or quality sleep.

The ideas in this book are based in holistic thinking and natural medicine, meaning they focus on the whole body and trust its inherent ability to prevent and overcome illness and disease. You *can* take care of yourself. The emphasis is on health, on life. You were born with everything you need to be healthy. If you eat well, sleep well, get exercise, find fulfillment, and nurture optimism, you may not need aspirin, sleep aids, antianxiety medications, or stimulants. Nothing could be simpler. Balance is our natural state. You are born healthy, and if you follow your body's guidance, you will stay that way.

Unlike anything man-made, your body, when balanced, knows what's best. It doesn't need you at the controls. We would all do better if we stepped aside and allowed our bodies to take the wheel. In terms of survival—living long, healthy, and strong—your ancient instincts know best.

This will work. Sleep is one of life's most simple pleasures and one of its most powerful functions, and it's immediately available here and now.

Part One: The Hows and Whys of Insomnia

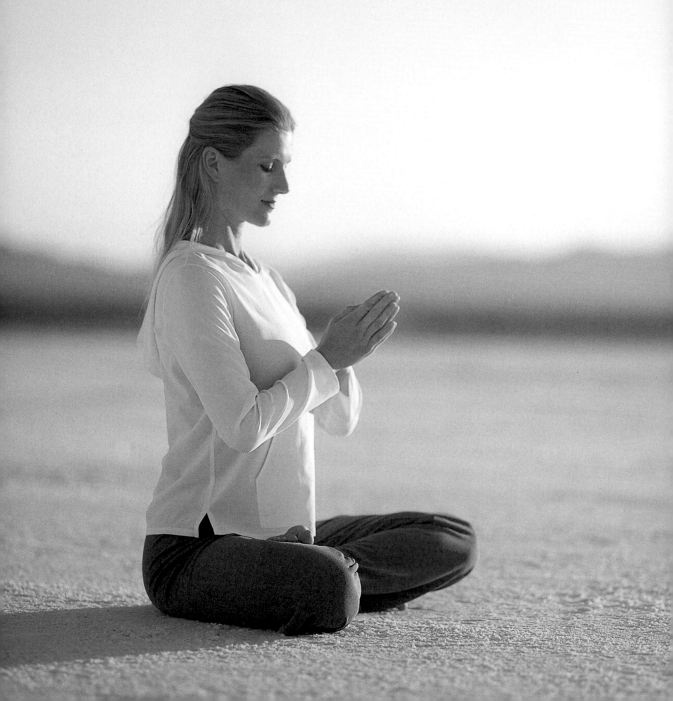

1

Truths about Sleep

Is sleep a mystery to you?

If you answered "yes" to this question, don't worry. Sleep is one of the least understood of physiological processes. Even most scientists and researchers in the field of sleep disorders don't completely understand it. However, one thing we do know is that sleep is critically important to quality of life and overall well-being. On sleep-deprived mornings, you may greet the day expecting the worst. Your performance at work, your personal relationships, and your mood may suffer.

Sleep is both a fundamental need and the ultimate elixir for health, yet it's one of the most undervalued human needs in our society. Instead of looking for more sleep, we seek other sources of energy, such as coffee. When we do try to sleep better, we go for over-the-counter and prescriptive cure-alls whose long-term side effects may only make things worse. We dash from one quick fix to the next, be it a sleep-inducer or a stimulant, treating the symptoms and not the cause.

This strategy overlooks the most effective, least expensive solution out there, and that is lifestyle modification. The broad goal of this book is to get you back in touch with your body's natural rhythms—specifically, those that govern the realm of sleep—and to return you to that place where your body functions on its own, waking and sleeping in an unbroken rhythm, never requiring conscious intervention on your part. I hope you get to the point where your body is so balanced and well-rested that any temporary disturbance to your sleep patterns will cause no more trouble than a quickly dissipating ripple causes on the calm, smooth surface of a pond. Now that's the sort of balance we're looking for.

THE QUEST FOR SLEEP

When was the last time you felt genuinely well rested without having taken a sleeping pill, glass of wine, or beer to help you sleep? When did you last feel genuinely awake and refreshed without a cup of coffee or an energy bar? While most people can recall an occasional good night's sleep, it's hard to find those who can say they sleep well every night. Few say they aren't tired.

The National Sleep Foundation's 2002 "Sleep in America" poll suggests that many health issues that have become part of the North American lifestyle, from obesity to stress and rage, stem in part from inadequate sleep. Poll results show that as many as 47 million adults say they're not getting enough sleep to feel alert. Roughly 10 million Americans rely on the multi-million-dollar-a-year prescription sleep medication industry, and that doesn't include those who use over-the-counter sleep aids or herbal remedies to help them sleep. When the National Sleep Foundation polled primary care physicians in 2002, 97 percent believed that inquiring about patients' sleep habits should be an essential part of a routine checkup, yet about half of these physicians reported occasionally, rarely, or never screening their patients for sleep problems. Thus, they're relying on you, the patient, to bring it up. The problem is, most people take sleep for granted and don't realize that lack of quality or quantity sleep can affect their health. In this same poll, 95 percent of primary care physicians agreed that insomnia can result from lifestyle imbalances rather than true medical causes.

8 SIGNS YOU'RE NOT GETTING ENOUGH ZZZZs

Think you're getting enough sleep? If you regularly find yourself doing any of the following, chances are you could use more rest.

* Abusing the snooze button.

* Waking up exhausted.

* Using coffee, tea, cola, or some other highly caffeinated beverage as a crutch to physically get you through the day.

* Sleeping profoundly and for hours as soon as you leave home base. (For example, using a weekend in the country to catch up on sleep.)

* Catching a cold or flu every time you take a break.

* Feeling inexplicable depression or irritation.

* Experiencing a lack of mental acuity, motivation, commitment, or the ability to focus.

* Having the eternal sense of being shortchanged, or feeling that you don't have enough of anything.

Need More Sleep?

Research suggests that most people do best with between 6½ and 8 hours of deep sleep in one stretch at night, though there are some who are fine with less. It's highly individual.

However, just because you get sufficient sleep in terms of quantity doesn't mean you're getting it in terms of quality. Although you're in bed with your eyes shut, and for all purposes you're asleep for 6½ to 8 hours, you wake up exhausted. What happened? The cause could be physical—shallow breathing, stress, and nutritional deficiencies can challenge your body during the day, making you sleep less soundly at night. It could also be mental. Sleep, for you, may be a harried experience. Your dreams might be fragmented and filled with to-do lists, snippets of conversations, wild daydreams, or worries. The function of these dreams, during the only downtime of your day, is to empty your cluttered head. It's not exactly rejuvenating.

And contrary to popular belief, you can't catch up on your sleep. If you think you can go all week on not enough sleep and then gorge on sleep on the weekends to make up for it, you're wrong. Research suggests that you can get away with a bad night every now and then, but two or three in a row fall into an irretrievable hole of sleep loss. However, even though you can't catch up, you *can* start over if you're making a change for good.

Remember, with chronic sleep deprivation, the only person denying you is yourself. Some people just resist sleep. They don't let their bodies shut down. They won't give in and rest. To rest might seem lazy, a cop-out, or a waste of time. And even when they give in and try to go to bed early, they can't for the life of them get more than their standard shortfall of rest. So instead, they stay in high gear for up to 20 hours a day, and say that they, like Einstein, only need to sleep for 4 hours.

WEAN THE BEAN

There's nothing wrong with enjoying a good cup of coffee. But there is something sad about needing one, two, or five cups, especially every day. In Chinese medicine, coffee is often referred to as "false chi," or false life force. Wouldn't you rather be driven by an authentic life force—your very own strong and sustained vitality?

Don't panic. You probably don't have to give up coffee forever, and you don't have to go cold turkey. Just be aware. And remember, you won't need it as much when you take care of yourself. Here are six simple steps to weaning yourself from the bean.

1. Substitute decaf for caffeinated coffee, or fill your cup with half decaf and half caffeinated coffee. But don't kid yourself. "Decaffeinated" coffee does contain caffeine—about 4 mg per cup. And it still contains the same acids, volatile oils, and tannins as caffeinated coffee. Drinking decaf does not give you license to drink twice as much.

2. Drink fewer cups each day. Start by drinking one fewer cup each day for a week. Each successive week, cut out your last cup of the day.

3. Try substituting green drinks, such as green tea, which provide a great energy boost, in place of coffee. (Go easy on the sugar, though. Some of them can have 2 tablespoons of sugar per serving.)

4. Replace your cup of coffee with a cup of tea or a glass of freshly blended fruit or vegetable juice.

5. Nurture your new habit as much as you relished your coffee one. Make a ritual of your cup of tea or your freshly blended juice. Buy accoutrements like a beautiful kettle, a juicer, or a blender. Sit down to drink your tea or juice with the paper or a book in a sunny corner. Sometimes it's not the thing itself we miss so much as the ritual around it.

6. Remind yourself of coffee's other negative effects: bad breath and brown teeth. In addition, drinking coffee makes you sweat.

This is usually denial in every sense of the word. Strung out by four daily cups of coffee and hectic schedules, these people just can't tell they are tired anymore. They deny that they need more sleep because they think they function fine without it, while in truth their day is like a racecourse marked by pit stops offering quick pick-me-ups to keep them going: sugar, caffeine, sugar, caffeine.

You may recognize yourself here. If you do, have compassion for what you're dealing with. You've made the first step toward balance by beginning to educate yourself about health and well-being. The most important thing you can do is be honest. Ask yourself, "Do I need more sleep?" If you have chronic difficulty falling asleep or staying asleep, or you suffer from chaotic sleep, you are missing an ingredient vital to mood, performance, and physical health. The answer is yes, you do need more sleep.

PHYSICAL CONSEQUENCES

Not getting enough sleep can have many physical effects on our bodies other than fatigue. Related disorders include depression, arthritis, lupus, weight gain, type 2 diabetes, and hypertension. In addition, the chemistry of stress and fatigue can cripple your immune system, leaving you unable to ward off illness.

A sleep-challenged immune system may manifest itself as acne, allergies, asthma, frequent colds and flus, conjunctivitis, infections, excess mucous production, rashes, sinusitis, styes, and more. This may be one reason why people under chronic stress acquire autoimmune-like tendencies, catching every cold that crosses their path and developing sensitivities or intolerances to things like lactose, wheat, and yeast, as well as developing seasonal and environmental allergies.

When many of my sleep-deprived patients first come to me, they are fighting one illness or another for most of the year, drowning their symptoms in cold medicines and covering up their fatigue with stimulants instead of nurturing themselves back into balance. This is no way to live. The problem is compounded by the fact that an imbalanced immune system overreacts and wears itself down, becoming less effective when you really need it. Instead of protecting you against disease, your own system can make you more prone to illness. Long term, if you don't give your immune system a chance to regenerate, you may risk facing serious disease.

YOUR MENTAL HEALTH

Lack of sleep and an inability to manage stress are closely intertwined. When you're tired and not performing your best, you become judgmental and irritable. You feel ineffective and unable to deal with life's challenges.

Losing sleep is unsettling. Many who suffer from sleep disorders feel emotionally unstable, unable to cope, and incapable of living fully. Some feel less well equipped for life's challenges, less able to avail of its gifts, and less emotionally available for friends and family. People often fall into a place of chronic not-enoughness. It's called "scarcity thinking"—the idea that you never have everything you need. Not enough time, not enough energy, not enough help, not enough money, not enough fun. This mindset sets us up for a life of deficiency. It also invites compensatory excess: not enough to drink, so I'll have another; not enough shoes, so just one more pair; not enough to eat, so time for a treat, just to make myself feel better.

Does this sound familiar? Even the most positive person can fall into a mindset of deprivation that starts with insufficient rest.

Lack of sleep can also affect you on a spiritual level. When you have energy, you feel like you have limitless opportunity. When you don't sleep or feel well, you think your options are limited. Feelings of chronic scarcity can cause a slow deterioration of the spirit as you begin to see yourself as deficient. You become someone who can't be stretched any further.

CAN YOU AFFORD A BAD NIGHT'S SLEEP?

Feeling tired isn't the only adverse effect of a restless night. According to the National Sleep Foundation's 2002 "Sleep in America" poll, people who don't get enough sleep also report:

* eating more than usual;

* difficulty getting along with others;

* difficulty making decisions; and

* making more mistakes.

WHY NOT POP A PILL?

Sleep aids, whether over-the-counter or prescription, can be used judiciously as short-term solutions to the occasional restless night. However, they're not intended for long-term use and may have side effects. In fact, rebound insomnia can occur as a result of growing dependence on such medications. This is true not only for prescription medication but also for some over-the-counter meds and some herbal preparations. Sleeping pills, natural or synthetic, treat the symptom, but they don't usually address the cause.

Such measures keep you from getting to the root of the problem and doing the work it takes to establish balance in your life. They may be psychologically as well as physically addictive or have negative side effects associated with extended use, such as agitation, constipation, dizziness, headache, and nausea.

One of the most significant adverse effects of sleeping pills is the damage they can do to your confidence. You only resort to taking a pill when you don't really believe in your body anymore or trust yourself to get to sleep on your own, and you feel you can't waste time trying.

Free from Sleeping Pills

If you use sleeping pills, ask yourself why. You might be living life in a way that prohibits sleeping naturally. You're so wired at night, you can't relax. Maybe you could unwind on your own, but you don't even take the time to try. Unwinding only takes 5 minutes if you do it purposefully. (Watching television doesn't count as unwinding.) If you have a 5-minute wind-down, you have a potential solution. Here are some of my favorite ways to let your guard down before going to bed:

* Practice a breathing exercise (see page 32).

* Nourish a peaceful hobby, like drawing or writing in a journal.

* Brew a nice cup of chamomile or passionflower tea, and let it steep while you close your eyes and open your senses to the aroma of the herbs.

* Soak in a warm aromatherapy bath.

* Give yourself a foot reflexology massage. With your thumb, massage back and forth along the bottom of the arch of your foot. Next, apply pressure to the tip of your big toe for 20 to 30 seconds. Switch feet. Start over. This can add hours to a night's sleep!

* Perform a 5-minute meditation (see page 41).

* Perform the Savasana yoga pose (see pages 153 and 154).

To wean yourself off sleeping pills (check with your doctor first), consider substituting one of the natural remedies that tends to have fewer side effects. In general, you should take herbal or other natural sleep aids on an as-needed basis. Try not to assume that you need the extra help every night. Give your body a chance to fall asleep on its own.

YOUR SLEEP ACCOUNT

Sleep is like an investment. Give it value the way you would a new car, a stock portfolio, an expensive suit, or a new home. Keep a mental sleep log just as you keep track of important purchases, your weight, or your checkbook. Make sleep a vital aspect of good health, a priority. One way to do this is to create a system of deposits and withdrawals and be sure to keep it balanced in your favor.

The first step toward balancing your sleep account is to be aware. We all do things that aren't in our best interests. Take a look at your daily activities and ask if they're working well for you, then identify the specific habits you suspect may get in the way of sleep. Look at your eating tendencies and at the way you handle emotions and stress. Do you use caffeine or stimulants? Do you skip meals, including breakfast? Are you too much a people pleaser, saying yes to things you simply don't have time do to? These are hard habits to break. These are also sleep "withdrawals."

Balance the things that deplete your energy stores, such as drinking too much caffeine, working excessive hours, or running around after your kids, by replenishing your mind and body with a relaxing activity: 5-minutes of meditation, 20 minutes of yoga, writing in your journal, knitting, or taking a warm bath. These are sleep investments, or "deposits." If you don't make enough deposits, you'll bankrupt your energy. One, two, or three nights without quality rest will empty your account.

"TO YOU" LIST

- Take a moment at the end of every day this week to track your sleep routine in a journal. Write down everything you've done for the previous 24 hours and how it affected you physically and mentally. Each day, make sure to include:

  Diet: Meals, snacks, and drinks; include the time of consumption and the effect it had on your body and well-being.

  Exercise: What type? When?

  Mood: Any significant mood moments? What were they, when were they, what happened? Are any of them related to food or exercise, or to specific people or parts of your life?

  Energy: When was it up? Down? Any marked fluctuations? Always low? (Don't confuse a caffeine buzz with energy.)

  Sleep disruptions: Do you have problems falling asleep? Staying asleep? Nightmares? Poor quality of sleep? Do you awake hungry or anxious? What goes through your mind while you try to get back to sleep?

- Take note of any epiphanies you've had regarding sleep. Do you sleep especially well in certain climates? When you're on holiday? At a hotel? Do seasons affect your ability to sleep? In what environments do you sleep well, and what of those environments is missing from your home? Write down all your sleep successes and consider trying them again.

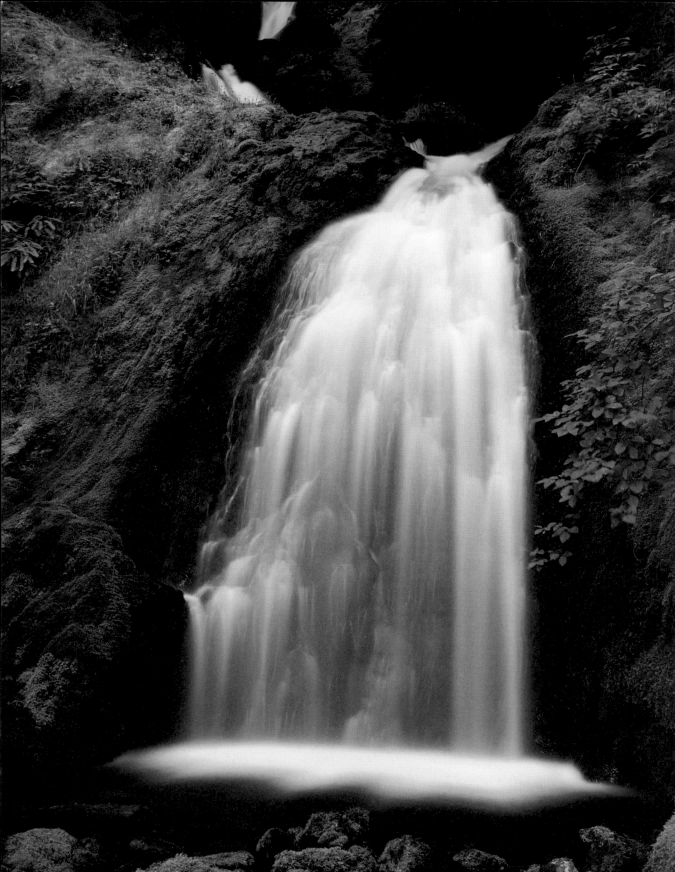

2

The Roots of Insomnia

What makes you feel alive?

The first step toward discovering what's keeping you up at night is to rule out more serious causes of insomnia, including Alzheimer's disease, anxiety, asthma, cancer, drug-related problems, heart or kidney disease, Parkinson's, sleep apnea (periodic cessation of breathing), heavy smoking, and thyroid conditions. Work with your physician to rule out these possibilities. However, if you have been diagnosed with any of the conditions listed above, the solutions outlined in this book will still benefit your health and your sleep. But keep in mind that the suggestions are not intended to be a cure-all for any or all diseases. It's imperative to consult and work with your family physician whenever you embark on any major lifestyle changes.

Take a look at other tangible forces that may be waking you up. Maybe it's something obvious, such as jet leg, muscle cramps, or the fact that you've had too much caffeine—or maybe you just took a decongestant before bed. Most often, though, a combination of factors is triggering your inability to rest. For example, a nutritional deficiency (such as a lack of calcium or magnesium) that keeps you from getting into the deeper realms of sleep may cause you to wake at every sound and bump in the night.

In the vast majority of cases, the inability to sleep can be traced to underlying psychological and spiritual issues—the intangibles. Even if something from your outer environment wakes you up—like your snoring spouse—something in your internal environment, such as worrying about your job, may keep you from falling back to sleep. The mindset that allows you to be overcome by worry is indicative that there's something else going on, a deeper lack of connection. Somewhere, somehow, some aspect of your life doesn't fit with who you are or what you want.

In Chinese medicine, this basis of insomnia is often referred to as "disturbed shen," or an unsettled spirit. It's caused by a life out of balance or a disconnect with your heart's peace and desire. Disturbed shen may be expressed as anxiety or tension, dissatisfaction or indifference, feeling generally out of sorts, or as an inability or unwillingness to answer your own basic needs, including sleep.

We can change the things that cause disturbed shen, though. By addressing the causes of your insomnia, there's a good chance you'll find yourself slumbering soundly in the near future. It just takes a willingness to do the work to find the cause or causes of your unrest. Sometimes it's difficult to put an emphasis on the things that give you joy in life because you have feelings of unworthiness. Don't allow yourself to go there. Self-fulfillment and honoring yourself are wonderful sleep aids.

NOURISHING THE SPIRIT

A busy mind and an undernourished spirit can be obstacles to, among other things, cultivating restful sleep. As I mentioned earlier, disturbed shen indicates that on some level you're not taking care of yourself; some basic requirement is not being met. This could be a nutritional, physical, emotional, or spiritual need, or a combination of needs.

Disturbed shen signals a disruption of the mind/body connection. Knowing your body well, including what affects it and how, takes focused attention. Honoring that knowledge—in effect, doing what your body tells you to do—requires loyalty to health and wellness. If you're not in touch with your body, you're usually not in touch with your mind. If you're not in touch with your mind, you may be missing out on some of life's opportunities. Disturbed shen may be a result of living half-heartedly. We become unable or too indifferent to make health a priority. When we water ourselves down, neglect our natural gifts, settle for less than who we are, and give our power away, we may be living less than courageously.

Nurturing shen is about living with courage and living in balance. Going after the life of your dreams feeds your spirit. It gives you a glow. You can see the sparkle in people's eyes when their spirits are happy. Our spirits shine when we're in love with life, trusting its possibilities, and are healthy and living our dreams.

I can't stress enough the significance, in terms of health, of living wholeheartedly. In the process of reading this book, answering some of the questions it poses, and spending time with yourself, you will begin to name and define what's out of harmony in your life, and you will begin to put it back in place. You will rediscover what gives you joy and begin to give yourself more of it.

Living in the Present

A good way to begin aligning with your spirit (opening up your heart and honoring its intention) is to get into the present as much as possible, either through meditation exercises or just mindful intention. Too many people live their lives focused on the past or the future, which generally only serves to produce unnecessary remorse or anxiety. Although it's beneficial to learn from the past and be prepared for the future, strive to live life in the present. Once you're more directly focused on the here and now, ask yourself if you want to be where you are. Simultaneously, define what stands in the way of peace for you. What stands in the way of giving you more life?

This is not to suggest that you up and quit your job, leave your family, or move to another city, state, or country. Dissatisfaction is usually more about internal factors than external ones. Even if you don't love your job, it may have nothing to do with your reason for unhappiness. Life is full of compromises, and they don't have to make us miserable. Give yourself time to get through the layers concealing the real root of your unease. Find it and resolve it, or you won't be satisfied at any job, in any life. Small shifts in perspective can do more to give you peace than big changes in the material facts of life.

At the same time, consciously work to discover what gives you joy, and give yourself permission to do more of that. If you can begin to do more of the things that make you feel fulfilled, you will be more at peace with your efforts. We all have mundane tasks and obligations. When the areas of your life that matter are in place, life's innate challenges become much more doable.

Creating Your Own Reality

You can also help align with your spirit by creating your own reality. Spiritual, philosophical, and psychological mentors have taught that we create reality through our thoughts. What we think about is what we become. She who has stressful thoughts is a stressful person. He who has fearful thoughts is generally afraid.

It's hard to explain in scientific terms why this works. Part of it boils down to faith, but a lot of it can be illustrated by what amounts to quantum physics. We all have an ever-changing electromagnetic field of energy surrounding our bodies. Some people call these subtle energy fields and yes, they are subtle, but they're profound in terms of their implications.

The nature of your energy field is influenced by your interactions with other people, your surroundings, and your health, moods, and perceptions. When you focus on a thought, your mood changes the nature of that field as perceptibly as it does your physical body chemistry. That field—what some healers call an aura—increases your likelihood to attract more of the quality you emit. Like attracts like.

What we surround ourselves with is what we become. These are very powerful ideas. If you spend the day absorbing bad news and reacting to it, it will start to affect your energy and have an impact on what you invite into your life. If you focus on joy and abundance, imagine what may come your way. Attract a great night's rest by emanating feelings of peace and compassion. Foster an empowered thought, and see what comes of it. If the psychology of your life is not supporting peace, peace can't happen.

TRY A MEDIA FAST

Do you regularly watch the evening news or have the news on as background noise, such as when you're driving to work or cooking dinner? If so, don't underestimate how this constant flow of mostly gloom and doom may be affecting you. At the end of the day, you may not feel like you have any hope. You may be in a place of reaction instead of possibility. Your dreams may seem insignificant, your life, lackluster.

The media can be a very powerful tool. It can instruct, inspire, and inform. But it, like anything, should be consumed mindfully.

Try, for one week, or for as long as you can, to avoid the media completely. Don't watch television or movies and don't read magazines or newspapers. Use the time you would have spent soaking up the media's messages doing things that make you feel alive. If you usually read the paper every morning, listen to music or go for a walk instead. When you return to the news, magazines, movies, and television, take the time to notice how what you see, read, and hear affects you. Become selective. You have a choice about what you let through the filter of your mind and spirit. Turn the television off when there's nothing worth watching! Pick the headlines that will really serve you in some way.

I'm not saying you should turn a blind eye to your world. But you should be in control of your emotional state and have power over how you spend your time. This will help you steer through the world more peacefully.

Start by being aware of your thoughts. Pessimism can become so much a way of life that people don't even realize their insidious decline of spirit, especially when hopelessness is veiled as sardonic or sarcastic humor, a self-deprecating manner, or a kind of jaded sophistication.

Slight changes in your outlook can be hugely powerful. Speaking kindly of yourself and your life will give you a feeling of control and will increase your ability to make a positive impression on the world—and by that, I'm talking not only about your image, but also about your spiritual imprint. So instead of thinking about how much money you're going to save this year, think about how much rest you'll get. Envision a better life for yourself. Invite balance. You'll change your life and the lives of those around you for the better.

BALANCING YOUR HORMONES

Hormones such as serotonin and melatonin direct our circadian rhythms, the 24-hour biological cycles that guide our physiological functions, including when to eat, when to sleep, and when to wake. Governed by light, circadian rhythms emit the chemistry that helps you sleep when it's darker. So when the sun goes down, you should, too.

Serotonin affects our moods, encouraging feelings of happiness and calm. Serotonin is produced from an essential amino acid called L-tryptophan. You can raise your serotonin levels by eating right, exercising regularly, and making other healthy lifestyle choices, such as practicing stress-management techniques like meditation and focused breathing.

MELATONIN BOOSTERS

Because melatonin appears naturally in some foods, the United States Dietary Supplement Health and Education Act of 1994 permits it to be sold as a dietary supplement. Melatonin can be purchased over-the-counter and has been shown to be effective at helping some people sleep better. It's a fine short-term solution, but melatonin is only an effective sleep aid if low melatonin production is the cause of your sleeplessness. If you experience sluggishness or excessive unusual dreams after taking it, this may mean that your melatonin levels are fine and that a lack of melatonin is not the reason you can't sleep. You don't need more of it, so supplements won't help you.

If you *do* need higher levels of melatonin, it's best to support your body's own production of it; that way, you have a dosage determined by nature. If you eat well during the day, move your body, and take time to relax, you should be able to maintain healthy serotonin—and thus melatonin—levels. Think of the last time you went on a laid-back vacation to a destination like the ocean or the mountains, where all you did was exercise, eat well, chill out, and sleep. How did you sleep then?

Another way to encourage your body's natural melatonin production before you go to bed is to honor nature's rhythms. Signal bedtime with gradual darkness about an hour before you go to sleep by turning off any bright overhead lights and using subtler lighting from lamps. This mimics nature's nightfall, and makes more sense to your body than immediate darkness after absolute brightness. Make your surroundings support your body's coming down from the day, and let it ease into melatonin production. This honors and helps you reconnect with the rhythm of your life.

After nightfall, the body converts that valuable serotonin to equally valuable melatonin. Melatonin, produced by the pineal gland, oversees the circadian rhythm that determines our sleep cycle. Darkness is key to supporting melatonin levels. Within the 24-hour circadian cycle, our bodies react to daylight, darkness, and changes in melatonin quantities, with rising and declining awareness and body temperature.

Keeping serotonin levels healthy and balanced can help with melatonin at bedtime. But if you're out of balance or experiencing low serotonin levels during the day, your chances of having melatonin at night can be challenged.

Because hormones work properly with the circadian rhythms only when they're part of a balanced system, women, with their naturally undulating hormones, are twice as likely as men to have difficulty falling asleep or staying asleep, especially during pregnancy, PMS, or menopause. But anyone's hormonal boat is susceptible to mutiny. Our delicately balanced physical chemistry is quite easily disturbed by stress, diet, emotion, a sedentary lifestyle, and poor respiration.

The Stress Factor

Stress hormones impact body chemistry in a way that is unfavorable to rest. The stress response, dubbed the "fight-or-flight" reaction, absolutely does not want the body to rest; it wants to prepare the body for battle. This stress response is an old, old friend that we can thank for our lives. But it's so old a friend that it's often inappropriate to the way we live our lives today. We're wired for a fairly primitive set of challenges: lions, tigers, and bears, for example. We're not wired to sit at a desk battling foes like computer crashes, the international marketplace, or bills. We're not wired to exercise patience in traffic. These contemporary foes don't require physical responses from us. If anything, they require stillness at a time when every instinct we possess tells us to move.

If we did move, we would help to dissipate those stress hormones properly. But because we are so stationary in most of our daily routines and challenges, there's an excess of those hormones coursing through our systems, causing stimulation, inflammation, and irritation everywhere they go.

So what can you do about stress? Start by looking at the way you manage stress. Instead of trying to avoid stress by limiting yourself and your opportunities, you need to learn to manage your response to stress. Be a person of possibility instead of a person of reaction. Prepare yourself on an emotional and physiological level for life and for stress. We can temper the fight-or-flight chemicals with behaviors that calm the body and the mind, support your inherent brain/body chemistry, and allow the circadian rhythms to balance.

Establish a Routine

One way to keep the fight-or-flight chemicals in check is to give your circadian rhythms a little positive reinforcement with a solid daily routine of waking times, mealtimes, exercise times, and bedtimes. Sticking to night and day patterns honors healthy hormone levels. Our bodies love habit, and it's one of the best things for combating insomnia. Begin to build a routine that works with your life—one that includes waking time, sleeping time, downtime, and doing time.

Our biological need for routine may well be one of the reasons every culture traditionally held rituals of prayer, washing, and change of attire around mealtimes, before bed, and upon rising. Until recently these were social cornerstones, important for psychological, social, spiritual, and physiological reasons. Not only did they mark the sanctity of the activity of eating or sleeping, they were also a signal to the brain to switch gears.

DON'T FEED ANXIETY

What you choose to eat and drink can do a great deal to enable or discourage sleeping well. Consistent mealtimes are important for healthy sleep chemistry and blood sugar levels. Avoiding foods high in sugar and making a promise not to skip any more meals can prevent a hypoglycemic wake-up call at 3 A.M.

Other dietary factors to be aware of are caffeine and other stimulants, often disguised in soda, ice cream, chocolate, coffee, tea, and some medicines and dietary supplements.

Alcohol is another sleep deterrent. In fact, the relationship between alcohol and sleep is a deceitful one. If you think alcohol helps you fall sleep, you've been misled. There's nothing like passing out for getting some quick shut-eye, but alcohol-induced sleep is simply not of a very high caliber, due to the hypoglycemic wake-up call I mentioned above. (To say nothing of the frequent need to urinate on nights when you've consumed excessive alcohol.) You may fall asleep quickly on nights when you've been drinking, but you probably wake often and early and have poor quality of sleep.

BREATHE DEEPLY

Another key component to establishing a healthy sleep chemistry is paying attention to your breath. Most of us breathe shallowly. Quick and shallow breathing, or forgetting to breathe altogether, are respiratory patterns that, as far as our brain is concerned, signal fear, action, or anger, and set off a stimulating stress response. On the other hand, breathing deeply puts you in a place physiologically where it helps to curb anxiety. When your respiration slows down, your body naturally produces a nonstress chemistry.

Aromatherapy can do the same thing. It acts on the limbic system (the part of your brain that regulates stress levels, heart rate, blood pressure, and breathing) to get the body into a state of relaxation. In 1995 the *Lancet* published a double-blind study on the use of a lavender oil diffuser that was as effective a sleep aid as *benzodiazapenes*, a group of sedative drugs that include valium. So while you're inhaling deeply and exhaling fully, slowly, and gently, put a little lavender essential oil on your clavicle and enjoy the double benefits! (See page 142 for tips on using essential oils safely.)

TEMPER ANGER AND ANXIETY

Keeping your emotions in check will also help you manage stress more effectively. Of course, that doesn't mean you should temper joy. Rather, try not to fuel your anger and anxiety. Refrain from stressful encounters after a predetermined hour in the evening, well before bedtime. This includes having discussions about difficult issues, paying bills, or making tough decisions.

If you've had stressful encounters all day and it's difficult to get them out of your system, go for a walk at the "stress-free hour," and visualize all the things that

BELLY BREATHING

Allowing yourself to breathe well from your belly offers the opportunity to always be present, mindful, and moving toward greater peace and harmony. It's a way to reconnect with the here and now. Practice breathing from your belly throughout your day—from the time you get up in the morning until you go to bed at night. If you make belly breathing a part of your life, you're guaranteed to experience greater feelings of peace and calm.

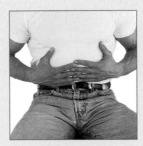

FIG. 1

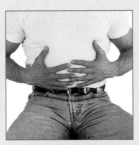

FIG. 2

✳ Begin by sitting comfortably in a chair. Be sure to sit all the way back, square on your sit bones, with a long spine touching the backrest of the chair. Place your feet slightly wider than hip-width apart, and place your hands on your abdomen, slightly interlacing the ends of your fingers. (Fig. 1) As you breathe, feel how your stomach feels against your hands. Feel the rise and fall of your diaphragm.

✳ Now, relax your head and neck, sit up tall, and release your shoulders. Feel your shoulder blades open up to your back and fall down toward your spine. Inhale deeply, feeling your fingers separate as your diaphragm presses lower into your abdomen. (Fig. 2) Inhale comfortably; be relaxed with your breath. Hold for a brief moment and begin to exhale. Release your breath evenly, feeling your stomach become smaller as your fingers begin to interlace again. As you near the end of the exhalation,

engage your abs and squeeze all the air out. Hold briefly and begin to inhale again. Sit in this position and continue to breathe deeply until you feel your body relax and settle. Maintain a tall spine and keep your head, neck, and shoulders relaxed at all times.

✳ As you develop a deeper pattern of breathing, feel your fingers pull in toward your spine as you exhale. Engaging your abs to press all the air out is very therapeutic, as it helps flush the lungs of toxins.

✳ As you inhale, use your hands and fingers to gauge how even your breath is. Feel your hands expand on your belly in equal intervals from inhalation to exhalation. Feel your diaphragm press down into your abdomen, creating more space for your lungs to expand and bring in vital oxygen. In addition to being therapeutic, working your breath this way helps tone your abs.

make you feel full of life. If you're so tired and down at that moment that you can't think of anything that makes you happy, try thinking of a beloved hobby, a good friend, or a great time in the past, and indulge in the happy associations you have. Remind yourself that you are the same person now as you were then, and invite that joy back into your life.

When you do have difficult conversations, no matter when they are, try to put drama aside. Don't be afraid to take a break. And always, always, remember to breathe from your belly.

CREATING BOOKENDS

In today's world, we've gotten away from letting our bodies rest—we've gotten away from practicing downtime. Too many of us wake up and head immediately to the phone, the computer, or the office. We go straight from resting to *doing*, or worse, we try to go straight from performing staggering physical and mental feats to trying to sleep.

The solution to all of this doing is to create bookends to your day. Bookends reinforce a routine that allows for downtime. While consistency is half the battle for sleep patterns, having a schedule for downtime is the other half. Do less. Be more. Allot at least 10 hours in a row, every day, to quiet time—approximately 7 of which will be spent in bed, sleeping. Give yourself an hour and a half every morning upon waking to relax and meditate with a cup of tea, go for a walk, stretch, or get some other form of exercise. Give yourself an hour and a half every night before going to bed where you refrain from stressful conversations and stimulation, including watching TV. Instead, just enjoy some relaxing music. This is a good time to dim the lights!

Before you protest and say, "I don't have an hour and a half in the morning! I can barely get started in time as it is. I'll end up sleeping less if I do this!" try to take a leap of faith. You will sleep better if you allow for downtime. Six and a half quality hours of sleep are better than seven and a half of scattered rest. But you should not have to cut any hours from your sleep time. Don't try to pack it in with all the other things you are *doing*. There's no reason you can't make this change simply by prioritizing. It may take a while to get it right and do it consistently. It may take some time to prioritize other areas of your life. Just trust it, and try. Your life activities will reshuffle on their own.

This is about creating a routine that revolves around your well-being, not around your earning capacity or your duties vis-à-vis other people. But it's also about having fun again! Give yourself time to play, time to be creative and open. Have courage. Widen your definition of yourself and your world.

REST ROADBLOCKS

Can't figure out what's keeping you up at night? Check out the following glitches to getting a good night's sleep to see if any may be affecting you.

❋ **Temperature.** Your room is either too hot or too cold.

❋ **Light.** There's too much light in your room. If you have bright streetlights outside, buy window blinds or wear an eye mask. Even the light from a digital alarm clock can be too stimulating for a good night's sleep.

❋ **Electromagnetic fields.** The energetic fields emitted by cell phones, computers, electric blankets, electric clocks, and other electronics stimulate the brain. These gadgets produce a noise that you can't consciously hear, but your body can, and it may be keeping you awake. Buy a good old-fashioned alarm clock (run by battery), charge cell phones in the next room, treat yourself to a cozy comforter, and make sure that all other electronics are turned off or unplugged.

❋ **Allergies.** The histamine response of allergies, set off by dust, mold, or other environmental stressors, can discourage a good night's rest. If you wake up with itchy eyes, congestion, or shortness of breath, try allergy-proofing your room

with allergenic bedding. Clean your room regularly with a HEPA filtered vacuum cleaner. If you still have symptoms, treat yourself to a HEPA air filter.

❋ **Noise.** Invest in some earplugs to block out the neighbor's barking dog (or the neighbor!).

❋ **A messy room.** Your sleep environment should be calming, uncluttered, and clean. Do not combine work and sleep space.

❋ **Pain or discomfort.** Stretch gently before bed. Take a hot bath to relieve muscle soreness. If your knees ache, lie on your back and prop a pillow under your knees so your legs are gently bent. If you have carpal tunnel syndrome, exercise your hands with Chinese Harmony Balls before bed. You could also practice self-massage (see page 144).

❋ **General comfort.** Maybe your bed's simply not very inviting. One of my patients slept an additional hour a night after she bought a comforter, just because the extra coziness made it so much harder to leave the bed.

"TO YOU" LIST

- This week in your journal write down:

  — Key stressors, such as work, relationships, and food.

  — Ways you fool yourself into not sleeping.

  — The things that wake you up or keep you up at night.

  — An action plan for resolving those issues.

- Start a new schedule. Pick one sleep deposit and add it into your existing routine. Make sure it's one thing you can and will do without fail. For example, promise yourself you will belly breathe first thing in the morning before you even get out of bed and last thing at night before you go to sleep. Other suggestions you might try include:

  — Make time for a nutritious breakfast. (See Chapter 5 for inspiration.)

  — Set a sleep routine that allows for about 7 hours of sleep.

  — Schedule downtime for yourself at the end of every day, even if it's just a 5-minute walk, to help yourself switch gears.

  — Promise yourself you won't skip meals.

- Use floor or table lamps for soft lighting. At a certain time in the evening, say around 8:30, turn off the bright overhead lights and turn the lamps on. In another half-hour, dim the lights. You could even sit by candlelight for 5 to 10 minutes. This will encourage melatonin production before you hit the sack.

- Play some beautiful, relaxing music that will set your mental stage for sleep.

- Create a balanced to-do list. Every time you "do" something, "be," as well. For every errand you run or task you complete on your to-do list, make the next obligation be to yourself and your blueprint for balance. For example, if you go to the grocery store, treat yourself to sitting quietly with a lit scented candle or perform self-massage with some body oil.

- Keep a gratitude card. Write down 10 positive things about your life, and read them aloud to yourself three times a day.

Part Two: Solutions for Sleep

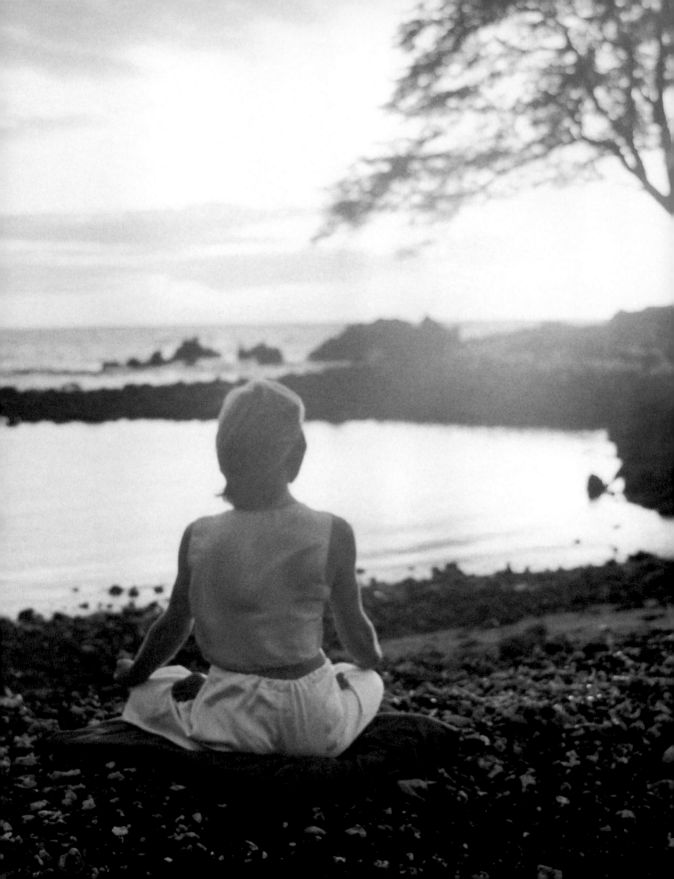

3

Finding Peace

Does your brain have a mind all its own?

If you're suffering from sleep problems, there's a good chance that your mind is at the root of your problems—meaning you're focusing too much on the negative aspects of your life and not enough on the positive ones. And somewhere along the line, your mind has interrupted your body's natural ability to nurture you with deep sleep. Some part of your life—whether physical, mental, emotional, or spiritual—is inhibiting rest. The process of healing discussed in this book will return you to your balanced and rested self and will encourage you to examine every area of your life to find the roots of your predicament. The idea of the sleep account, which I discussed in Chapter 1 (see page 20), can also be applied to the awareness work I'll be teaching you to do. Begin by asking yourself: What makes me feel stronger and more full of potential, more positive and alive? Also look into what detracts from that: What is making withdrawals on your spirit?

Focusing on the positive takes mental discipline, but the rewards are tremendous. Half the battle against mental restlessness, pessimism, and anxiety is won just by becoming more optimistic.

Yoga and meditation, both of which will be discussed later, are critically important means to this end. Both yoga and meditation are built on the idea of mindfulness, the ability to focus the mind on the breath, a thought, or an affirmation. Both enhance the mind/body connection, and both are great long-term solutions to insomnia. Practicing mindfulness and bringing awareness to the breath are the most effective ways to regain and maintain balance—psychologically, physiologically, and spiritually.

When I talk about meditation, I'm not referring to being in a trance. Meditation can be thought of as the same thing as focused contemplation, prayer, introspection, or taking a quiet moment. You can also meditate on emotions such as joy or gratitude—doing so will help you to better experience and recognize those feelings. Meditation, or mindfulness, is about being present, focused, and centered. It's about disciplining the mind, enhancing mental clarity, and boosting energy. One of meditation's greatest gifts is that it allows you to create mental and emotional space. If you nurture that space and maintain it, no one person or amount of work or stress can take it away from you.

In addition to priming you spiritually for optimism and possibility, meditation also works on your body chemistry to make happiness and balance more accessible for you physiologically. In combination with attention to the breath, meditation lowers the production of stress hormones in the body, encourages an alkaline environment that discourages disease, and also lowers blood lactate, which is associated with anxiety.

Shallow breathing—which is how most people breathe—causes the release of stress hormones such as cortisol. Relaxed, deep breathing keeps this from happening. Breathing exercises can also keep you focused on the present, so you may feel less anger and anxiety over the past or the future.

There are many kinds of meditation. You can meditate anywhere, for any amount of time. Meditation works on many levels. With meditative breathing practices (such as belly breathing; see page 32), you'll establish a positive chemistry for sleep. Meditation also helps relieve stress, which allows your body to absorb the nutrients essential for good health.

MEDITATION EXERCISES

If you practice yoga and meditation regularly, you'll find that you're able to relax more quickly. Ease—rather than jump—into meditation, and create a setting and ritual around meditation. For example, light a scented candle and play some meditative music. Eventually, these props will work to set off a Pavlovian reaction in your brain. Your body will know that relaxation is to follow and will begin to settle in before you even start.

You can meditate in many different ways. Find a time and place that are right for you. The best way to incorporate meditation and mindfulness into your day is to schedule it into your bookends (see page 33), with a morning and an evening practice. On top of that, practice mindfulness exercises throughout your day. This combination of activities will truly put you in a completely different state of mind in as little as a few days.

Meditation for the Morning

To prepare for morning meditation, sit cross-legged on the floor on a sofa cushion, folded blanket, or firm pillow. Sit forward on the cushion so your hips fall slightly forward and your spine remains vertical and erect; keep your neck and shoulders soft. Position your hands and arms so they're comfortable. Take a few moments to think about the present moment.

Inhale deeply through your mouth, concentrating on releasing your breath completely. Inhale deeply again, taking in as much air as possible, filling every inch of your lungs. Exhale slowly and evenly through your nose, engaging your abs and pulling in toward your spine as you press all the air out. Continue this breathing pattern for 2 or 3 minutes. On each inhalation, concentrate on the here and now. During each exhalation, focus your mind on awakening your spirit and energizing your body.

Meditation for the Evening

Begin this meditation by lying down on a blanket. Extend your legs about hip-width apart, hands and arms slightly away from your body, palms facing up. Relax, then inhale deeply through your nose. Feel your belly expand and your chest rise. Exhale slowly through your mouth. Inhale deeply again, taking in as much air as possible, then exhale slowly.

On each inhalation, breathe into an area of discomfort, starting with your feet and moving up your body toward your head. On each exhalation, allow your breath to carry the tension and stress away from the area of focus. Continue this breathing pattern for as long as it takes you to relax your body and mind.

Meditation on the Go

The following are short meditation practices that you can perform anytime, anywhere. You can do them sitting up or lying down, with your eyes open or closed.

✳ **Belly breathing.** (See page 32.)

✳ **Visualization.** This form of relaxation can help you turn your most heartfelt desires—health, abundance, and even sleep—into reality. To perform visualization, picture in your mind's eye the image of whatever you desire, and hold this image. If your greatest desire is to sleep, try picturing a place of peace and calm. Use your belly breathing to align your body and mind with your peace-giving inner landscape to promote feelings of peace and tranquility.

✳ **Affirmations.** These positive statements are your personal reminders of your potential, validations of who you are and what you want out of life. Their function is to keep you centered and motivated. Affirmations can focus on long-term issues—such as "I am healthy" and "I am talented." Or you can change them according to each day's needs—such as "I will ace today's presentation." Write your affirmations down and then read them out loud at least twice a day.

✳ **Yoga breath.** Close your eyes and inhale slowly through your nose for 4 counts, making sure you fill your belly, then your back, and finally your chest with air. Hold the breath for 2 counts. Exhale slowly, through pursed lips, for 8 counts. Repeat this breath 5 times.

"TO YOU" LIST

- This week in your journal, write down all the positives in your life.

- Rub a lotion with a calming scent, such as lavender, on your skin after you shower.

- Make a cup of decaf herbal tea. As it steeps, close your eyes and inhale the fragrant tea from the cup. Sip the tea slowly and meditate on its taste and smell.

- Treat yourself to a simple daily aromatherapy massage. Put a dab of essential oil on the inside of your wrist, below your pinky. (See page 142 for tips on using essential oils safely.) This area is known as your heart channel, and it is associated with anxiety and restlessness. Rub the lotion in gently and enjoy its smell as you go about your day.

- Surround yourself with peace props—tokens of things for which you feel blessed—such as keepsakes from family members, a photo of your favorite place, or pictures of friends. Take a 5-minute break every hour to reflect on these things and feel grateful for them.

4

Exercising for Body and Mind

Is your life an out-of-body, out-of-control experience?

I like to tell my patients, "Exercise only on days when you eat." In other words, do it every day. You don't have to run 10 miles, seven days a week. Just do something daily that you enjoy and that works your whole body. If you're healthy, it's easier to feel good about life. Exercise, we know, has everything to do with strength and vitality. The major benefits of physical fitness include optimum respiratory and circulatory function. Working out is second to none in protecting cardiovascular health and can be the primary factor that separates people who don't die from heart disease from those who do. It boosts the immune system by supporting white blood cell activity and encouraging natural killer cell function, a primary defense against diseases such as cancer. People who exercise regularly catch fewer colds, and when they do catch something, the illness is more likely to pass quickly through their systems. Weight-bearing exercises prevent osteoporosis.

In general, exercise keeps the body strong and supple, increases lean muscle mass, and burns fat. And the more lean muscle mass we have, the better. Around age 40, we begin to lose an average of 6 pounds of lean muscle mass every decade. That means that by the time you're 70, you'll have lost about 20 pounds of muscle. By building your store of lean muscle, exercise—particularly weight-bearing exercise—keeps you younger longer. Weight training is also essential for increasing insulin sensitivity in the body, which means it helps prevent two of America's most serious epidemics: obesity and diabetes.

FITNESS AND SLEEP

In addition to all those great health benefits, movement can also significantly improve your quality of sleep. After all, exercise, even walking, is one of the best things you can do to manage tension. It lowers stress hormones, a key culprit in insomnia. Mindful movement in combination with deep breathing supports the parasympathetic nervous system, which puts our bodies in a state of relaxation and aids in supporting optimum production levels of serotonin and melatonin.

Exercise also does wonders for the spirit. There's peace in the knowledge that we've done something for ourselves on any given day. Many insomnia patients confess to using sleepless moments to daydream, problem solve, and address their goals, or to stress out about what they're not getting done in their lives. There's something about going to bed knowing that, having exercised that day, you took care of yourself and lived more fully. That self-respect translates into peace of mind. Exercising is a way of taking charge of your health.

By having you focus on your body for a block of time every day, exercise also strengthens your mind/body connection and creates a support system that works against mental busyness. By putting you in a good place emotionally and physiologically, movement will motivate you to make other healthy choices.

EXERCISE IN A NEW LIGHT

If you hate gyms, despise work-out contraptions, don't have time to find the nearest swimming pool, and can't be bothered with fitness accessories in an already cluttered home, then the program in this book is perfect for you. Exercise doesn't have to be so formal. After all, exercise is about moving in a variety of ways all day long. Chances are, if you're giving life your all, you're already moving. Getting kids dressed and sending them off to school, running daily errands to the store and post office, and even preparing for a vacation can feel like running an obstacle course. This daily workout could be enough to keep you in shape, if you did it with attention to your breath, posture, and muscle function.

Begin to notice how you use your abs for everything from sitting down or sweeping the floor to taking a book down from a high shelf. Take breaks every half-hour to go for a brisk 5-minute walk, even if it's just in your office building or to the corner and back. Stretch slowly and breathe deeply into tension spots. Your body works very hard for you. Give it a little positive feedback for all it does. Give it what it needs to do its job.

What counts is to make the most of your daily activities. Engage in conscious movement, movement that you do for yourself and your health. Be aware of how you breathe and how you carry yourself in everything you do. Chances are, once you begin to face your body and its abilities this way, exercise will begin to seem a little less out of reach.

Breath of Life

Breathing is nonnegotiable—obviously, you have to breathe to live. Breathing supplies our muscles and organs with oxygen, the fuel they need to function. Inhaling deeply and exhaling completely with every breath does much more than keep us

ONE STEP AT A TIME

If you can't get past the idea of working out, keep this in mind: Every little thing you do to move more and move mindfully during the day can make a difference to your health. Even just one hour a week of walking lowers your risk of heart disease. So walk to the post office or the corner store instead of driving there. Buy a pedometer, record the number of steps you take in a day, and do what you can to increase it. One of my patients lost 95 pounds in a year and a half just by parking further away from the entrance to the grocery store and eating well. When she first turned the pedometer on, she was walking about 2,500 steps a day. Now she walks about 12,000. Walk for 10 minutes every morning and every evening, and you'll begin to feel on fire with purpose.

alive, though. It helps maintain our physical and mental health. And yet breathing, like sleep, is something most of us take for granted.

Conscious breathing practices during exercise and during every activity of the "doing" portion of your day will not only improve your physical and mental performance, they will also help boost your mind/body connection. Deep breathing is critical for keeping cortisol (the primary stress hormone in the body) balanced. When cortisol is out of balance along with DHEA (an adrenal hormone), vitality, muscle tone, and sex drive can be affected.

Voluntary deep breathing, as in meditation, yoga, and tai chi practices, complements aerobic exercise and does so in a body-friendly way.

In general, when engaging in aerobic exercise, it's best to breathe deeply and regularly through your nose. Whether you're swimming, walking, or jogging, make your inhalations last as long as your exhalations. Remember that your lungs aren't located in your collarbones; they extend to the bottom of your rib cage, and they fill the front and the back of your body. When you breathe, make use of all that space and fill it with air. At the same time, make sure your breathing is relaxed. Panting and gasping with your mouth wide open will leave you exhausted, which is the last thing you want.

The most important thing to remember about breathing well is that you can do it anywhere and anytime. Make it part of your lifestyle.

The Benefits of Yoga

Yoga is an essential part of my sleep program for both the physical and mental benefits it provides. Stretching relieves tension in the muscles, while breathing oxygenates the body, revitalizing your every fiber. Yoga practice is all about letting go of the tight grip that you maintain on your life for every other moment of the day, dropping your barriers and shields, and getting into your body, moment by moment. It's deeply satisfying, energizing, and relaxing. _

If you can't get your mind around the idea of yoga, think of it as calisthenics or stretching. Whatever you call it, the yoga positions, or *asanas,* are a wonderful way to help you come back to center and get your breathing back in balance. Yoga is an incredible tool for fitness for athletes of all levels.

BREATHING EXERCISES

Many of us do not breathe to our full capacity, which decreases the amount of oxygen in our bodies. This deficiency contributes to fatigue, stress, irritability, anxiety, and many sleepless nights. Developing positive breathing habits is essential to maintaining a balanced body and mind, increases our ability to focus our minds, helps to calm our bodies, and lessens the stressful effects of everyday life. An awareness of your breath is an essential tool to help increase your body's ability to heal itself.

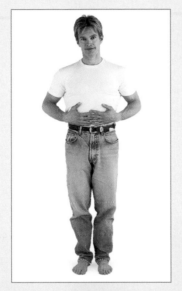

FIG. 1

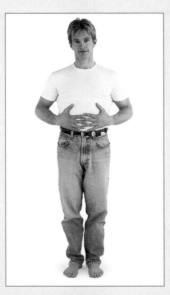

FIG. 2

✴ Spread your feet slightly apart, and place your hands on your abdomen, interlacing just the ends of your fingers. (Fig. 1) As you continue to breathe, feel how your stomach feels against your hands. Feel the rise and fall of your diaphragm.

✴ Now inhale deeply, feeling your fingers separate as your diaphragm presses lower into your abdomen (Fig. 2); be relaxed with your breath. Hold for a moment and begin to exhale. Release your breath evenly, feeling your stomach become smaller and your fingers begin to interlace again.

✴ As you near the end of the exhalation, engage your abs and squeeze all the air out. Hold briefly and begin to inhale again. Maintain a tall spine and keep your head, neck, and shoulders relaxed at all times.

✴ As you develop a deeper pattern of breathing, feel your fingers pull in toward the spine as you exhale. Engaging your abs to press all the air out is very therapeutic, helping to flush your lungs of toxins.

MORNING YOGA PRACTICE

Each morning is a fresh opportunity to set a healthy tone for your whole day. This simple yet powerful yoga practice can help you begin each day energized and centered by using deep breathing to oxygenate your muscles and focus your mind. Morning is the perfect time to practice exercises that open up your body, create balance and aware- ness, and energize your spirit. Practice this sequence every morning and you'll begin to experience a more relaxed body and a calmer, more focused mind.

To do the complete routine, perform each posture in the sequence as it's shown, from start to finish. Hold each posture for 5 long, even breaths, and then move to the next posture.

To access the deeper effects of each posture, you can practice each pose in sequence or individually, holding for up to 1 minute with attention to comfortable, relaxed breathing. You could also practice this routine in the evening to prepare for a restful, restorative night of sleep and to let go of daily stress and deeply relax.

Keep in mind that proper positioning is very important in all yoga postures to achieve the intended benefit. In most people, one side of the body is stronger than the other. Be aware of how your body feels, and check your alignment.

MOUNTAIN POSE

Mountain Pose is the starting place for all standing poses. It's called Mountain Pose because in it you stand tall, upright, and steady. Done correctly, this upright posture reduces stress, and when performed properly, it can increase your focus.

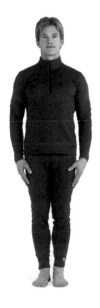

FIG. 1

Stand tall with your feet parallel and close together. Spread your toes out. Extend your arms down along your sides, fingers pointed toward the floor. Reach up tall through your head, looking straight ahead. Breathe deeply and consistently.

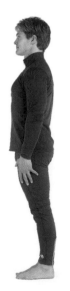

FIG. 2

To feel the posture and find the proper position, stand with your legs firm. Tighten your knees slightly and firm your buttocks. Keeping your stomach strong, lift your chest, spine, and neck straight up, as if a rope was pulling you skyward through the center core of your body. Breathe. Hold this posture for 5 long, even breaths. If you are practicing this pose individually, hold for up to 1 minute with attention to comfortable, relaxed breathing.

Note: Balance your weight evenly between your heels and toes.

Variation: If you're a beginner, start with your feet spread apart slightly and your heels and back firm against a wall.

MOUNTAIN POSE WITH ARMS OVERHEAD

Mountain Pose with Arms Overhead is a great pose for people who spend too much time sitting down. This posture helps relieve tension in your upper body and expand your breath capacity.

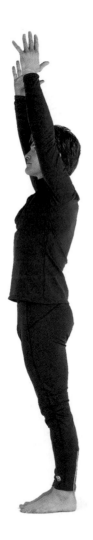

From Mountain Pose, exhale, raising your arms overhead, hands shoulder-width apart, fingers reaching skyward. Relax your shoulders and reach as tall as you can. Breathe. Hold this posture for 5 long, even breaths. If you are practicing this pose individually, hold for up to 1 minute with attention to comfortable, relaxed breathing.

Note: Don't scrunch your shoulders up as you reach. Relax your neck and feel your shoulders falling back and down.

Variation: For beginners, try this pose against a wall.

STANDING FORWARD BEND

In this posture, your spine stretches deeply and lengthens your hamstrings, which has numerous physical benefits. However, my purpose in including this exercise here is the calming effects that forward bending can offer your body and mind. This posture helps calm your nervous system by slowing your heart rate and rejuvenating your spinal column. Perform this posture anytime you feel the need to unwind.

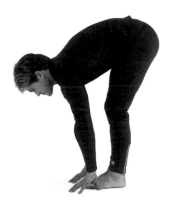

FIG. 1

From Mountain Pose with Arms Overhead, exhale and bend your knees slightly as you bend forward, placing your hands alongside your toes. Keep your back straight and long.

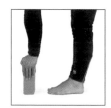

CLOSEUP DETAIL

If you cannot reach the floor with your hands or your hamstrings are too tight, use a yoga brick as an extension of your arms. This will allow you to extend your legs straight without bowing at your waist. If you don't have a yoga brick, use a big, firm book, or a stack of books. You want about 9 inches of height (maximum) for this prop, depending on your flexibility.

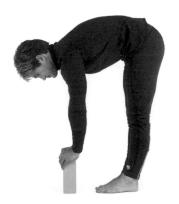

FIG. 2

Keeping your legs strong, extend out through your waist, straighten your legs, and allow your upper body to fold forward. Breathe. Use the brick for support or keep your knees bent until you feel comfortable and confident that you can reach the floor with your hands without straining. This posture is meant to be relaxing and calming; don't force the posture, or you'll eliminate the benefit. You should be able to breathe evenly and comfortably in this posture. Hold this posture for 5 long, even breaths. If you are practicing this pose individually, hold for up to 1 minute with attention to comfortable, relaxed breathing.

Variation: For beginners, start with your feet shoulder-width apart. As your flexibility increases and the pose becomes more comfortable, move your feet closer together until your heels and big toes are touching.

PLANK POSE

In this posture, you'll begin to strengthen the core of your body while creating support and mobility in the joints of your legs and arms. In Plank Pose, your wrists strengthen and stretch, creating positive mobility. When performing this pose, concentrate on balance between your hands and feet—the only parts of your body that touch the floor.

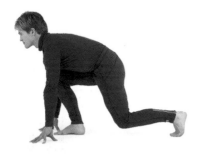

FIG. 1

From a Standing Forward Bend, inhale, then exhale, bending your knees, dropping your buttocks, and flattening your hands on the floor. Step back with your left foot, then your right, into an extended push-up position. Breathe.

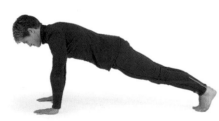

FIG. 2

Your hands are directly below your shoulders. Your feet are together, toes tucked under. Once you've moved into the posture, inhale and tighten your legs slightly. On the exhalation, reach through your arms, pressing firmly with your hands. Keep your shoulders relaxed and down away from your ears. Keep your stomach strong and firm, your neck soft, and look down slightly in front of you. Breathe evenly and deeply. Hold this posture for 5 long, even breaths. If you are practicing this pose individually, hold for up to 1 minute with attention to comfortable, relaxed breathing.

Note: Feel that your body is like a plank of wood. Imagine that you could draw a straight line from your head to your heels. Don't allow your hips to sag.

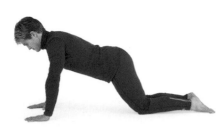

FIG. 3

If you have less arm strength, relax your knees down to the floor, keeping your arms strong.

Note: Don't fall back toward your legs. Your arms should still be stacked directly under your shoulder joints. You should feel as if you're holding yourself up by your hands and arms.

Variation: If you're a beginner, you can keep your feet spread slightly for more balance and control.

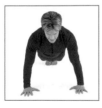

OVERVIEW

Proper positioning is very important in all yoga postures to achieve the intended benefit. Most people find that one side of their body is stronger than the other. Be aware of how your body feels, and check your alignment. Make sure you're stacked evenly from the right to the left side, and from front to back.

PUSH-UP POSE

Here you'll support your entire body on your hands and toes, strengthen your arms, develop powerful wrists, and tone your abs. Make sure you concentrate so you perform this posture correctly. When done properly, this posture can help relieve lethargy.

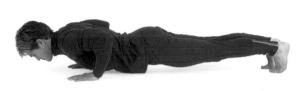

FIG. 1

Still in Plank Position, inhale. On the exhalation, lower your body toward the floor until you're about 6 inches above it. Keep your elbows tight to your body and your stomach strong and firm. Balance your weight evenly between your hands and toes. Maintain a long, firm body. Look down, slightly in front of you. Breathe. Hold this pose for 5 long, even breaths. If you are practicing this pose individually, hold for up to 1 minute with attention to comfortable, relaxed breathing.

Note: Your hands should be directly alongside your chest, fingers at your armpits.

Option: If you're a beginner, you can keep your feet spread slightly for more balance and control.

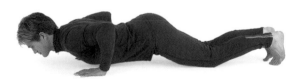

FIG. 2

If you have less arm strength, relax your knees down to the floor, keeping your arms strong. Your buttocks will elevate slightly, so focus on balancing the weight of your body evenly between your hands, knees, and feet. Breathe.

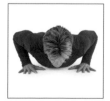

OVERVIEW

Be aware of how your body feels, and check your alignment. Make sure you're stacked evenly from the right to the left side, and from front and back.

UPWARD FACING DOG POSE

This posture is best known for stretching, strengthening, and rejuvenating the spine. It also helps to expand your chest and lungs, giving you more cardiovascular capacity.

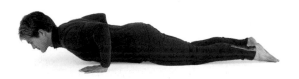

FIG. 1

From Push-Up Pose, exhale and release your entire body to the floor. Move your hands down to alongside your waist, elbows tight to the sides of your body, and lay the tops of your feet flat on the floor. Look forward.

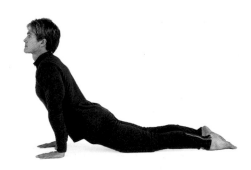

FIG. 2

Spread your feet about hip-width apart. Inhale. On the exhalation, pull your trunk forward and raise your head upward, pressing firmly with your hands and fully extending your arms. Breathe. Keep your legs firm and strong, and lift your knees off the floor. Push your chest forward and up, completely stretching your spine and thighs. Reach tall through your arms and keep your buttocks tight. Relax your shoulders down your back and away from your ears, creating space for additional length in the pose. Breathe deeply and evenly. Hold this posture for 5 long, even breaths. If you are practicing this pose individually, hold for up to 1 minute with attention to comfortable, relaxed breathing. To release the pose, bend your elbows and release your torso to the floor.

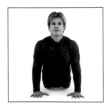

OVERVIEW

Be aware of how your body feels, and check your alignment. Make sure you're stacked evenly from the right to the left side, and from front to back.

DOWNWARD FACING DOG POSE

Most of us have seen this pose performed by countless pets. Downward Facing Dog is the most beneficial pose in the yoga repertoire—the pose of all poses. Done consistently, this posture can relieve numerous ailments, including fatigue and headaches. This pose stimulates blood flow to your head and chest, which rejuvenates brain cells and slows your heart rate. This pose also helps tone your legs, arms, and abdomen.

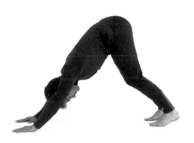

FIG. 1

Lie flat on the floor, keeping your feet about hip-width apart. Position your hands alongside your chest. Inhale. On the exhalation, press your palms into the floor and raise your torso up, straightening your arms. Drop you head toward your feet, push back, straighten your elbows, and extend your back. Your hips rise to the sky as you begin to press through your legs and extend back from your arms through your shoulders. With your knees slightly bent, begin to press back through your heels. Relax your neck and release your shoulders back. Feel as though your shoulder blades want to touch one another in the middle of your back. Keep your feet and hands pointing straight ahead. Hold this posture for 5 long, even breaths. If you are practicing this pose individually, hold for up to 1 minute with attention to comfortable, relaxed breathing.

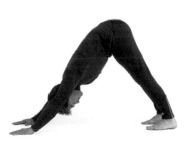

FIG. 2

Once you feel comfortable performing this pose, or if you have more flexibility, begin to straighten your knees and press firmly back through your heels. Remember to relax your shoulders. Breathe.

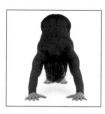

OVERVIEW

Be aware of how your body feels, and check your alignment. Make sure you're stacked evenly from the right to the left side, and from front to back.

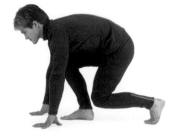

FIG. 3

To release the pose, on an exhalation bend your knees and drop your hips toward the floor. Walk your feet forward to your hands, keeping your knees bent and slowly raising your torso up to Mountain Pose. Breathe.

STANDING FORWARD BEND

To maintain the calming effect of this practice, let's continue by repeating the Standing Forward Bend. Some instructors believe that if you hold this position for at least 2 minutes, you can help relieve depression. Now that your body has warmed up and you're working with your breath, we'll move more deeply into this pose.

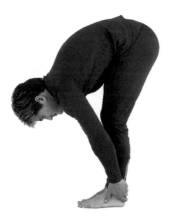

FIG. 1

From Mountain Pose, inhale, then exhale and bend slowly forward from your waist. Lightly grasp your ankles with your hands. Keep your knees slightly bent, your back long and supple. Keep your neck relaxed. Breathe.

Note: Don't force the stretch. Keeping your knees bent allows you to comfortably set the posture properly. Lead with your chest on the forward bend. Keep your back straight; fall forward from your waist.

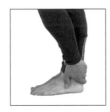

CLOSEUP DETAIL

Your hands should grasp your ankles for support, not to pull your torso down. If this is uncomfortable, reach your hands toward the floor alongside your feet.

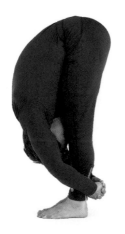

FIG. 2

When you feel ready and you can do it without straining, inhale and on the exhalation, begin to straighten your legs. Your hands should remain lightly grasping your ankles—or, if you feel confident, you can wrap them around the backs of your ankles. You can also keep your palms on the floor alongside your feet. Breathe. Hold this posture for 5 long, even breaths. If you are practicing this pose individually, hold for up to 1 minute with attention to comfortable, relaxed breathing.

MOUNTAIN POSE WITH ARMS OVERHEAD

To find our centers and realign ourselves, we come back to this position as a point of focus and stability. Use this position to feel the calming effects on your body and mind and to feel your breath as you inhale and exhale.

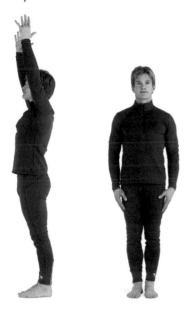

FIG. 1

From standing Forward Bend, inhale. Leading with your chest, reach long through your arms and raise your torso up. As you come to standing reach your arms overhead, extend, and exhale, slowly dropping your arms to your sides.

FIG. 2

Stand tall with your feet together, heels and big toes touching. Keep your legs active and strong. Reach tall through the crown of your head, keeping your neck and shoulders relaxed. Hold this posture for 5 long, even breaths. If you are practicing this pose individually, hold for up to one minute with attention to comfortable, relaxed breathing.

Note: Make sure to relax your neck and shoulders, releasing all tension away from your head.

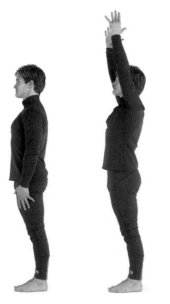

FIG. 3

Before we move ahead, feel the balance of the posture—that is, that all four corners of your feet are pressing firmly into the floor, that your legs are active, and that you're reaching tall through your waist. Relax your shoulders, allowing them to fall freely away from your neck. Breathe. Hold this posture for 5 long, even breaths. If you are practicing this pose individually, hold for up to 1 minute with attention to comfortable, relaxed breathing.

FIG. 4

Inhale and raise your arms up overhead, reaching tall through your hands and pressing firmly through your feet, keeping your legs active. Breathe deeply and evenly as you move to the next posture.

CHAIR POSE

Known to be a powerful pose, this posture helps to develop confidence and stamina. It also helps to evenly tone your legs and strengthen your ankles.

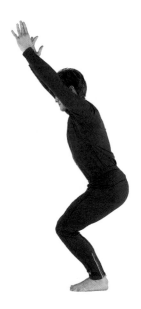

FIG. 1

From Mountain Pose with Arms Overhead and your feet together, exhale. Drop your upper body and hips toward the floor until your thighs are at a 45-degree angle to the floor. Extend long through your body, reaching tall with your hands. Breathe.

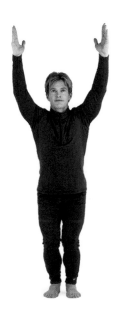

FIG. 2

Keep your neck soft and shoulders relaxed, dropping down your back. Your arms should be directly alongside your ears and your knees should be together. Breathe. Hold this posture for 5 long, even breaths. If you are practicing this pose individually, hold for up to 1 minute with attention to comfortable, relaxed breathing.

Variation: If you feel strong, drop your torso and hips lower to the floor. Try to lower your thighs parallel to the floor without straining or losing control of the posture.

STANDING FORWARD BEND

Transitioning through Standing Forward Bend gives you a moment to calm your body and mind. Perform this posture with purpose and intention. Your body is now much warmer, so use the added circulation to try to stabilize this pose by reaching long through your waist and spine, creating as much length through the back of your legs as possible.

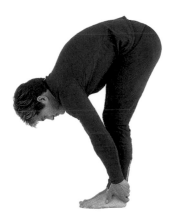

FIG. 1

From Chair Pose, inhale. On the exhalation reach long through your spine and waist, straightening your legs and allowing your torso to fall forward; reach your hands to your ankles. Lightly grasp your ankles with your hands, keeping your back long and neck relaxed. Breathe. Hold this posture for 5 long, even breaths. If you are practicing this pose individually, hold for up to 1 minute with attention to comfortable, relaxed breathing.

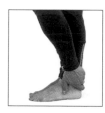

CLOSEUP DETAIL

Your hands should grasp your ankles for support, not to pull your torso down. If this is uncomfortable, reach your hands to the floor alongside your feet.

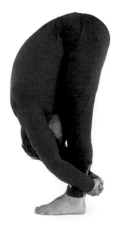

FIG. 2

When you feel ready, and without straining, inhale. On the exhalation, begin to straighten your legs. Your hands should remain lightly grasping your ankles. Or, if you feel confident, wrap them around the backs of your ankles. You can also keep your palms on the floor alongside your feet. Breathe deeply and evenly. Hold this posture for 5 long, even breaths. If you are practicing this pose individually, hold for up to 1 minute with attention to comfortable, relaxed breathing.

PLANK POSE

As you repeat this posture in the sequence, use this position to calm your breath and focus on body alignment.

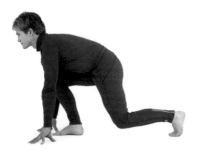

FIG. 1

From Standing Forward Bend, exhale, bend your legs, and step your left foot back and then your right. Be sure your hands are directly under your shoulders and shoulder-width apart.

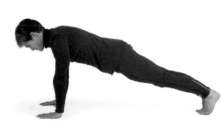

FIG. 2

Position your feet together, toes tucked under. On the exhalation, reach strong through your arms, pressing firmly with your hands. Keep your neck and shoulders relaxed. Breathe. Keep your stomach strong and firm, your neck soft, and gaze down slightly in front of you. Breathe evenly and deeply. Hold this posture for 5 long, even breaths. If you are practicing this pose individually, hold for up to 1 minute with attention to comfortable, relaxed breathing.

Note: Keep you abdomen firm so you don't tip your hips.

PUSH-UP POSE

This posture involves concentration. As you repeat this posture, focus on your alignment and stabilize this pose for maximum benefit.

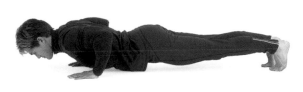

FIG. 1

On the exhalation, lower your torso toward the floor from Plank Pose. Be sure your elbows remain tight to the sides of your body, and keep your stomach and legs strong and firm. Balance your weight evenly between your hands and toes. Reach out and extend through your neck and head, keeping your shoulders relaxed. Maintain a long body in this posture. Hold this posture for 5 long, even breaths. If you are practicing this pose individually, hold for up to 1 minute with attention to comfortable, relaxed breathing.

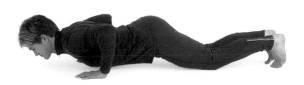

FIG. 2

If you feel fatigued in your arms and torso, move to the modified position with your knees on the floor to stabilize the pose. Keep your body long and press firmly through your hands with your elbows tight to your sides.

Note: Your hands should be directly alongside your chest, fingers at your armpits.

UPWARD FACING DOG POSE

As you move through this pose again, your body is warmed up, more relaxed, and open. Allow your body to reach long through your spine, letting your hips drop further to the floor and lifting your chest higher.

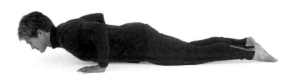

FIG. 1

From Push-Up Pose, inhale, then exhale, releasing your entire body to the floor. Move your hands alongside your waist, elbows tight to the sides of your body, and turn your toes back. Look forward. Breathe.

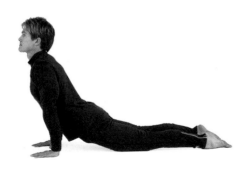

FIG. 2

Inhale. On the exhalation, press firmly through your hands and fully extend your arms. Reach through your chest and raise your torso up, extending through the top of your head. Keep your legs firm and knees off the floor, lifting your torso and thighs. Relax your shoulders down your back, creating space for additional length in the pose. Breathe deeply and evenly. Hold this posture for 5 long, even breaths. If you are practicing this pose individually, hold for up to 1 minute with attention to comfortable, relaxed breathing. To release the pose, bend your elbows and release your torso to the floor, to prepare for the next posture.

DOWNWARD FACING DOG POSE

Traditionally, this posture is considered a resting position, stimulating blood flow to the head and chest, rejuvenating the brain, and slowing the heart rate. Use this pose and your breath to rest before moving through the remainder of the sequence.

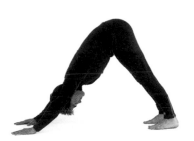

FIG. 1

In Upward Facing Dog, move your feet to about hip-width apart, hands alongside your chest. On the exhalation, press through your hands and raise your hips up to the sky, straightening your arms. Drop your head toward your feet, pushing back, straightening your elbows and lengthening through your back and waist. Press back through your heels, extending long through your arms and pushing back through your hips. Feel the length in the back of your legs and press firmly from your feet up through your waist, extending your hips as high as possible. Keep your neck and shoulders relaxed and press firmly and evenly through both hands. Breathe. Hold this posture for 5 long, even breaths. If you are practicing this pose individually, hold for up to 1 minute with attention to comfortable, relaxed breathing.

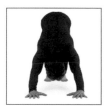

OVERVIEW

Find balance and comfort in your posture and use it as a moment of rest before you move on to the next pose. Breathe deeply with long, comfortable breaths. Keep your shoulders relaxed and your neck long.

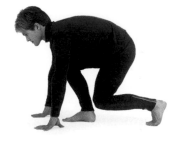

FIG. 2

To release the pose, inhale and walk your feet forward to your hands. Come to Forward Bend position, keeping your knees bent. Exhale, raising your torso to Mountain Pose, hands along your sides.

WARRIOR I

This pose is named after the mythic warrior Virabhadra. This posture helps to strengthen your legs, ankles, and spine, and it creates flexibility in your knee joints. It also helps to expand your chest for deeper breathing and tone your abdomen for better digestion.

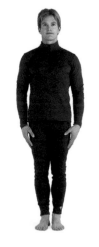

FIG. 1

Begin in Mountain Pose, with your hands at your sides.

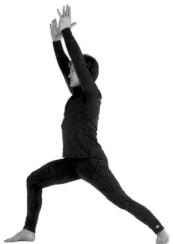

FIG. 2

Spread your feet 3 to 4 feet apart. Turn your right foot out to a 90-degree angle, and turn your left foot slightly in. Turn your torso to face out toward the toes of your right foot. Inhale. On the exhalation, bend your right knee so your thigh is nearly parallel to the floor. Lengthen your left leg and straighten your left knee. Breathe. Stretch your arms tall overhead; relax your shoulders down your back, keeping a soft neck. Hold this posture for 5 long, even breaths and then move to the other side, left leg forward and right leg back. If you are practicing this pose individually, hold for up to 1 minute with attention to comfortable, relaxed breathing.

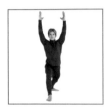

OVERVIEW

Your knee, hips, chest, and head should be facing directly out over your right foot. Breathe. Press firmly through each foot.

WARRIOR II

A variation of Warrior I, this posture helps to increase flexibility in your hips and knees. It also develops strength and endurance in your legs. In addition, this pose vigorously tones your entire torso and helps to increase your breath capacity.

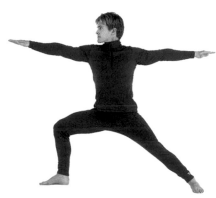

FIG. 1

From Warrior I, straighten your bent leg and turn your feet back to face straight ahead. Keep your legs spread 3 to 4 feet apart and lower your arms down to shoulder height. Reach long through your fingers. Turn your right foot out to a 90-degree angle and turn your left foot slightly in. Turn your head to face out toward your right hand. Inhale. On the exhalation bend your right knee so your thigh is nearly parallel to the floor. Lengthen your left leg and straighten your left knee. Breathe. Try to create a 90-degree angle between your thigh and calf.

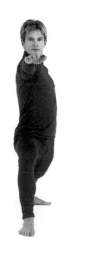

FIG. 2

Stretch your back leg firmly. Extend out through your hands, keeping your hips in line with your chest. Your knee should be facing directly out over your right foot. Stretch your arms wide and keep your hands at shoulder height. Relax your shoulders down your back, keeping your neck soft. Focus your vision over your right hand. Press firmly through each foot, reaching long through your back leg. Breathe. Hold this posture for 5 long, even breaths and then move to the other side, moving your left leg forward and your right leg back. If you are practicing this pose individually, hold for up to 1 minute with attention to comfortable, relaxed breathing.

PLANK POSE

As you transition through this posture again, concentrate on the height you create. Focus on your breath as you press up firmly through your arms, reaching as high as you can. Maintain a stable body and pay attention to length, reaching long through your legs and tall through the top of your head.

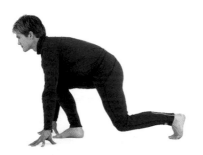

FIG. 1

From Warrior II, drop your hands to your sides and straighten your bent leg. Turn your feet forward, step your legs together, and move back to the front of your mat in Mountain Pose. Bend your knees and reach your hands to the floor, stepping your feet back behind you.

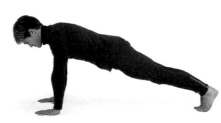

FIG. 2

Come to a comfortable, balanced position with your hands directly under your shoulders, Press up firmly through your hands, reaching your torso as high as you can. Keep your shoulders relaxed and your abdomen strong and firm. Your legs should be active, stabilizing the entire length of your body. Imaging that you could draw a straight line along the side of your body from head to toe. Maintain relaxed, comfortable breathing. Hold this posture for 5 long, even breaths. If you are practicing this pose individually, hold for up to 1 minute with attention to comfortable, relaxed breathing.

PUSH-UP POSE

Moving into Push-Up Pose at this point in the sequence will challenge your strength. As you repeat the pose, concentrate on deep breathing to access the power to perform this pose properly.

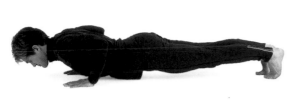

FIG. 1

From Plank Pose, exhale and lower your torso to about 6 inches above the floor by slowly bending your arms. Concentrate on lengthening your body to evenly balance your weight between your hands and feet. Maintain a firm, engaged abdomen and activate your legs to keep your torso from drooping toward the floor. Image again that you could draw a straight line along the side of your body from your head to your heels. Breathe. Hold this posture for 5 long, even breaths. If you are practicing this pose individually, hold for up to 1 minute with attention to comfortable, relaxed breathing.

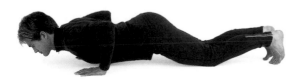

FIG. 2

If you are feeling tired and don't have enough strength to hold the pose, drop your knees to the floor in the modified position. Remember to keep your torso flat and extended, pressing firmly through your hands.

UPWARD FACING DOG POSE

As you perform this posture for the last time in the sequence, pay close attention and focus deeply on extension and length through your spine and chest. Allow your body to open up and accept the pose. Breathe deeply, creating extra length and space in your body on each exhalation.

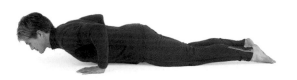

FIG. 1

From Push-Up Pose, release your torso to the floor, lying flat on your stomach. Extend long through your legs and be sure your hands are positioned alongside your body, even with your chest.

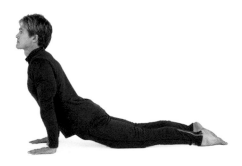

FIG. 2

On the exhalation, extend out through your head and begin to press your torso upward. Activate your legs and lift up through your chest as your head reaches skyward. Press firmly through your hands and, releasing through your lower back and abdomen, allow your torso to reach up tall. Keep a soft neck and relax your shoulders, feeling them fall down and away from your ears. Breathe. Hold this posture for 5 long, even breaths. If you are practicing this pose individually, hold for up to 1 minute with attention to comfortable, relaxed breathing.

DOWNWARD FACING DOG POSE

As I stated earlier in the sequence, this pose is meant for resting the body and mind—to create calm in your nervous system and to slow your heart rate. As you rest in this pose for the final time in the sequence, pay close attention to your breathing and how it affects your posture. On each inhalation, breathe into those areas of your body that may still feel tight. On each exhalation, reach into those areas and allow your breath to release that stiffness and tension.

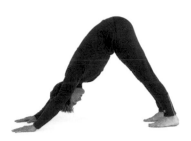

FIG. 1

From Upward Facing Dog, exhale and press back through your hands, lifting your hips high into the air. Reach long through your heels, extending through the back of your legs and up through your hips. Breathe deeply, pressing firmly through your hands and reaching back through your hips. Feel your shoulders release down and away from your ears and keep your neck soft, dropping your head down toward the floor. Breathe deeply and comfortably, allowing each breath to relax your body and mind even further. Hold this posture for 5 long, even breaths. If you are practicing this pose individually, hold for up to 1 minute with attention to comfortable, relaxed breathing.

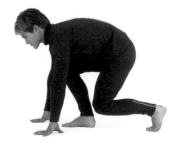

FIG. 2

To release the pose, keep your hands on the floor, exhale, and bend your knees, stepping your feet forward in between your hands. Take as many or as few steps as necessary. Hold yourself in the bent knee Forward Bend position.

STANDING FORWARD BEND

As you move into this final forward bend, focus more on existing in the posture than reaching the floor with your hands.

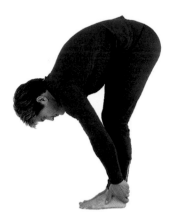

FIG. 1

From the bent knee Forward Bend position, grasp your ankles and reach long through your spine. Extend that length out through the top of your head. Relax your shoulders and neck and breathe deeply.

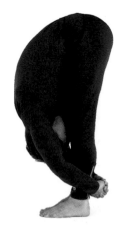

FIG. 2

On the exhalation, slowly begin to straighten your legs, reaching up tall through your hips and allowing your torso to fall forward toward your knees. Use your hands for support and do not pull yourself down. Let your breath create length in the pose, using each exhalation to lift through your legs and relax your torso. Feel that your body is hanging freely off the top of your hips. Maintain your balance by keeping your legs active and pressing firmly through your feet. Relax your neck and shoulders. Hunching forward will not help you bend further into the posture. Breathe deeply and evenly. Hold this posture for 5 long, even breaths. If you are practicing this pose individually, hold for up to 1 minute with attention to comfortable, relaxed breathing.

MOUNTAIN POSE

When you finish your yoga practice, you'll begin your day with calm intent. To set the tone for the day, you move into your final posture exactly where you began—in Mountain Pose. You finish with this posture to balance yourself and gain focus, to feel the energy flowing through your body, and to establish a strong awareness of your breath. Use this final minute or two to gain a positive understanding of yourself, your environment, and how you will move through the rest of your day.

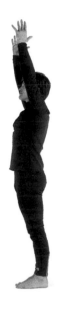

FIG. 1

From Standing Forward Bend, exhale and reach out long through your hands. Leading with your chest, lift your torso upward. Reach your hands up high overhead, extending tall through your body and maintaining a strong base with your feet. Breathe.

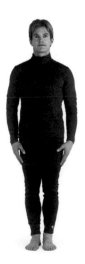

FIG. 2

Inhale. On the exhalation, slowly release your hands down to your sides, extending long through your fingers. Activate your legs, pressing firmly through your feet. Reach up tall through your spine, relaxing your abdomen but keeping your buttocks firm. Relax your neck and let your shoulders release down and away from your ears. Hold your body tall and steady. Breathe deeply, allowing calm to wash over you. Feel your breath and the rise and fall of your abdomen. Use this time to focus and deepen your awareness of the mind/body connection. Use your breath to expand this connection and establish your intent for a peaceful, fulfilling day.

EVENING STRETCHING AND RESISTANCE TRAINING

This evening practice concentrates on stretching and resistance training exercises with the use of the circleband—an oversize rubberband made specifically for use with these instructions. These types of exercises counteract muscle loss and increase your body's ability to burn calories. They also help relieve built-up tension and stress—factors that may prevent you from getting a good night's sleep.

Perform each exercise in the sequence shown. Complete the recommended repetitions and sets for each before moving to the next exercise. Be sure to pace yourself and concentrate on proper form, alignment, and breathing technique.

P.M.

CONCENTRATION CURLS

We think of bicep curls as exercises that tone our arms. In addition to shapely arms, curls also help keep your elbow and wrist joints strong, which helps to prevent chronic ailments such as carpal tunnel syndrome and tendonitis.

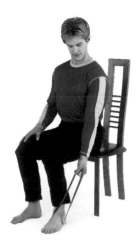

FIG. 1

Position yourself on your sit bones, squarely on a chair. Place your feet about hip-width apart and create a strong base with your feet. Stack your knees directly over your ankles. Take your circleband and place it under your left foot. Hold the other end of the circleband in your fingers, between your second and third knuckles. Extend your arm down and sit up tall. Use your right hand on your right knee to support your torso. Keep your spine erect and your shoulders square and level.

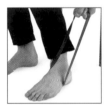

CLOSEUP DETAIL

Position the circleband under the arch of your foot, slightly forward and toward the ball of your foot. Always keep your feet square, toes facing forward.

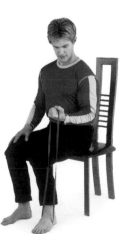

FIG. 2

Without lurching or jerking your body forward and back, slowly pull the circleband, focusing all your attention on the movement of your forearm and bicep. Pull upward until your forearm is parallel to the floor, hold, squeeze your bicep, and slowly release until your arm is fully extended. Repeat. The only motion should be your forearm swinging upward and the contraction and relaxation of your bicep muscle. Exhale as you pull and inhale as you release your bicep. Keep the movement slow and simple. The entire movement in both directions should last the length of an exhalation and inhalation. Repeat with your right arm.

Performance: Beginners—4 sets of 6 repetitions on each side
Advanced—6 sets of 12 repetitions on each side

Body logic: You might tend to lean into the movement on the pull and fall away on the release. Keep your body strong, and hold the core of your body up tall. Press firmly through the balls and heels of your feet to maintain your foundation. Don't hunch your back.

POWER CURLS

The principle behind power curls is to strengthen your arms while enhancing body coordination. The movement of this exercise is quicker than Concentration Curls but requires as much focus to be performed properly. It's a great exercise to elevate your heart rate and burn a few calories—and give you shapely arms at the same time.

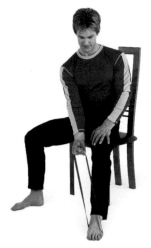

FIG. 1

Position yourself on your sit bones, squarely on a chair. Place your feet about hip-width apart, with your knees stacked directly over your ankles. Move your left foot out slightly wider than shoulder-width, extending your foot out just beyond your knee. Leave your right foot in place. Turn your left foot out at a 45-degree angle. Turn your torso to face your left toes. Place the circleband under your left foot; extend your right hand to hold the circleband. Sit up tall with your right arm extended down. Your left hand on your left knee supports your torso.

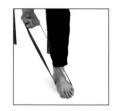

CLOSEUP DETAIL

Position the circleband under the arch of your foot, slightly forward and toward the ball of your foot. Keep your feet firmly planted on the floor.

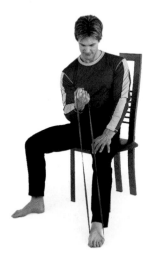

FIG. 2

Without lurching or jerking your body forward and back, pull the circleband firmly and quickly up toward your armpit; squeeze at the top. Pull as high as you can without moving your upper arm. Release quickly, and extend your arm completely. Focus all your attention on maintaining control during the movement. The only motion should be your forearm swinging upward and the contraction and relaxation of your bicep muscle. Exhale as you pull and inhale as you release your bicep. Keep the movement quick and controlled. Synchronize your breathing with the movement—exhale as you move up, inhale as you move down. Repeat with your left arm.

Performance: Beginners—4 sets of 10 repetitions on each side
Advanced—6 sets of 15 repetitions on each side

Body logic: You might tend to create excessive movement on the pull/release action with your upper arm. Keep your upper arm firm from your shoulder joint. Watch your elbow. If it rises and falls with the movement, try to hold your upper arm in against your side. Keep your body strong, and hold the core of your body up tall. Press firmly through the balls and heels of your feet to maintain your foundation. Don't hunch your back.

CONCENTRATION KICKBACKS

We'll complete the concentration circuit by focusing on the triceps muscles. This exercise involves isolating your upper arm by removing all leverage in a standing position. This movement helps to strengthen wrist and elbow joints along with enhancing the shape of your arm.

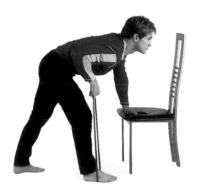

FIG. 1

Stand up, turn, and face your chair. Slightly bend your knees, reach down, and place your left hand on the seat of the chair. Spread your legs hip-width apart and stagger your legs, with your right foot forward, knee bent, and your left foot back, long and firm. Find a strong, stable stance that is comfortable for you when leaning onto the chair. Your feet remain firmly pressed into the floor at all times. Place the circleband under your right foot. Position your left arm, fully extended, hand flat on the chair directly under your shoulder joint. Keep your back flat and gaze straight ahead. Position your right arm at a 90-degree angle, your elbow tight to the side of your body, your hand slightly forward, pointing straight at your foot. The band should be almost vertical.

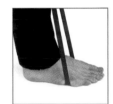

CLOSEUP DETAIL

Position the band directly under the ball of your foot. Press firmly through the heel, ball, and toes of your foot.

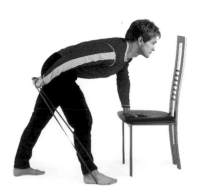

FIG. 2

Without leaning forward and down, slowly extend your right hand back toward your buttocks; keep your elbow tight to your body. Reach your hand back until your right arm is fully extended. Focus all your attention on the movement. Hold at the top, squeeze, and slowly release until your hand is pointing directly at your foot. Repeat. The only motion should be your forearm extending backwards and the contraction and relaxation of your triceps muscle.

Exhale as you reach and inhale as you release your triceps. Keep the movement slow and simple. The entire movement in both directions should last the length of an exhalation and an inhalation. Repeat with your left arm.

Performance: Beginners—4 sets of 6 repetitions on each side
Advanced—6 sets of 12 repetitions on each side

Body logic: You might tend to lean into the movement on the pull and fall away on the release. Keep your body strong and your left arm firm and pressing into the chair. Press through the balls and heels of your feet to maintain your foundation. Don't hunch your back. Keep your abs strong for better support.

POWER KICKBACKS

This exercise is very similar to Concentration Kickbacks, but you perform it faster. To increase the body coordination effect of this exercise, I've removed the chair to make it more challenging. Beginners can keep the chair and use the same setup as Concentration Kickbacks.

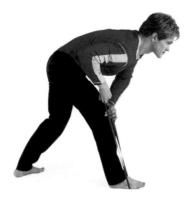

FIG. 1

If you want a more challenging exercise and a great way to really work your entire body, begin with your feet in the same position as in Concentration Kickbacks. Place your left hand on your right knee for support. Move your right foot ahead slightly, so your chin is even with your toes. Your right hand will now point down toward your knee and the circleband will be angled back slightly. Keep your back flat and focus your gaze a few feet in front of you. Maintain a strong core foundation between your feet and the support of your left hand. Engage your abs to stabilize your torso.

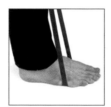

CLOSEUP DETAIL

Position the circleband directly under the ball of your foot. Press firmly through the heel, ball, and toes of your foot.

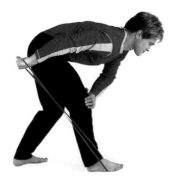

FIG. 2

Keep your right elbow tight to your body. Firmly and quickly reach your right hand back until your right arm is fully extended, then release back down, pointing your hand toward your knee. As soon as your hand comes to the starting point, press back with your hand. Squeeze at the top and release. Focus all your attention on the movement of your forearm. Exhale as you pull and inhale as you release your triceps. Keep the movement quick and controlled. Synchronize your breathing with the movement—exhale as you move up, inhale as you move down. Repeat with your left hand.

Performance: Beginners—4 sets of 10 repetitions on each side
Advanced—6 sets of 15 repetitions on each side

Body logic: In this position you'll experience a slight up-and-down movement in your torso. This is natural due to the motion itself. To work the core of your body, keep your back long and work to stabilize your core with your abs. Keep your left arm firm and pressed firmly into your right knee. Press through the balls and heels of your feet to maintain your foundation. Don't hunch your back.

STANDING TRICEPS EXTENSIONS

You'll complete the arm circuit with standing triceps extensions. We'll work the triceps again because they're the smaller of the upper arm muscles and sometimes they require more attention than the others. It's also easier to find your balance and posture using this movement when performing standing resistance exercises. This exercise will help to define your triceps and also tone and strengthen your abs and legs.

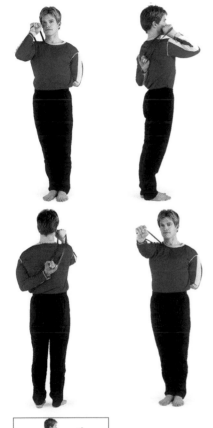

FIG. 1

Standing tall with your feet together, reach behind you with your left arm (as if you were going to scratch your back). Turn your palm so that it's facing up. Take the circleband in your right hand and reach back over your right shoulder. Grab the opposite end of the band with your left hand. Now reposition yourself so you're standing tall, with a long back, firm legs, and your feet pressing firmly into the floor.

FIG. 2

Bring your right upper arm up parallel to the floor, reaching your hand back over your shoulder. Your right elbow should be pointing straight ahead.

FIG. 3

Keep your shoulders square and parallel to the floor. Keep your buttocks muscles firm, legs reaching up strong. Your left arm should remain in a comfortable position. Keep in mind that your left arm and hand work to hold the band. Before you start, try pulling slightly on the band with your right hand to feel the tension. If you're a beginner and you feel unstable, spread your feet slightly apart to widen your foundation.

FIG. 4

Engaging your abs, extend your right hand forward, keeping your arm at shoulder height. Squeeze your triceps muscle and slowly release. Repeat. Your upper arm should remain stable and the only movement should be your forearm moving like a lever, forward and back, and the contraction of your triceps. Keep the movement steady and active; don't move too slowly. Exhale as you reach and inhale as you release back.

OVERVIEW

Engage your legs. Feel your feet pressing into the floor. Don't lean back; reach tall through your spine.

Performance: Beginners—4 sets of 8 repetitions on each side
Advanced—6 sets of 12 repetitions on each side

Body logic: In this position you'll have a tendency to lean forward and back. To prevent this, spread your feet slightly until you have strengthened the core of your body and found your balance. (Hint: Engage your buttocks muscles for better control.)

ANTERIOR DELTOID FLIES

We begin the shoulder circuit with Anterior Deltoid Flies. Flies work the front portion of your shoulder joint area—the small muscle group that helps you raise your arms up in front of you. These exercises help to strengthen the shoulder joints and enhance shoulder mobility by strengthening the smaller muscles that you don't use very much. The position of this exercise also helps to tone your abs, buttocks, and legs.

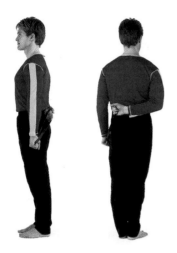

FIG. 1

Standing tall with your feet together, take your circleband in your right hand and reach it back behind you. Reach with your left hand and grasp the other end of the band. Your right arm will remain folded at a 90-degree angle, resting along your waistline. Extend your left arm straight down alongside your body. Your left hand should touch your thigh at the beginning and end of the movement.

FIG. 2

Keep your elbow and the palm of your left hand facing backwards (rotate your arm to the inside). Work to keep your arm rotated back to focus all the resistance on your shoulder. Press firmly through your feet, keep your legs strong, and engage your buttocks and abs. Reach tall through your spine, keeping your shoulders square and level.

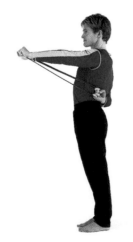

FIG. 3

Reach your left hand forward and up. Keep your left elbow firm, but not locked. Reach your hand to shoulder height, hold, and release back down to your side. Repeat. The movement should be even and smooth. Count to 2 as you lift, hold, and count to 2 to finish. Exhale as you lift and inhale as you release.

Performance: Beginners—4 sets of 8 repetitions on each side
Advanced—6 sets of 12 repetitions on each side

Body logic: In this position you might tend to lean forward and back. To prevent this, slightly spread your feet until you have strengthened the core of your body and found your balance. (Hint: Engage your buttocks and ab muscles for control.)

MEDIAL DELTOID FLIES

This exercise works the outside of your shoulder—the muscle that allows you to lift your arms out to your sides. If you want wider shoulders, this is the exercise for you.

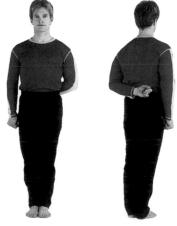

FIG. 1

Standing tall with your feet together, take the circleband in your left hand and reach it back behind you. Reach with your right hand and grasp the other end of the band. Your left arm will remain folded at a 90-degree angle, resting along your waistline. Extend your right arm straight down alongside your body. Your right hand should touch your thigh at the beginning and end of the movement.

FIG. 2

Keep the elbow of your right hand facing backward, your palm facing your thigh (rotate your arm to the outside). You'll feel this when you begin the movement. Work to keep your arm rotated back to focus all the resistance on your shoulder. Press firmly through your feet, keep your legs strong, and engage your buttocks and abs. Reach tall through your spine, keeping your shoulders square and level.

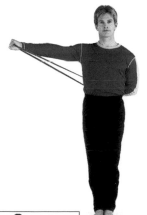

FIG. 3

Reach your right hand out and up to the side. Keep your right elbow firm, but not locked. Reach your hand to shoulder height, hold, and release back down to your side. Repeat. The movement should be even and smooth. Count to 2 as you lift, hold, and count to 2 to finish. Exhale as you lift and inhale as you release.

OVERVIEW

Maintain the proper position and keep your left shoulder from collapsing. If your support shoulder and arm collapse when you lift, reduce the height of the movement until you've gained more strength and increased your balance. Focus on keeping your shoulders square and level. Engage your buttocks and ab muscles for support. If you're a beginner, spread your feet apart slightly to establish a stronger foundation.

Performance: Beginners—4 sets of 8 repetitions on each side
Advanced—6 sets of 12 repetitions on each side

Body logic: In this position you might tend to lean away from the movement to gain leverage. To prevent this, spread your feet slightly until you have strengthened your core and found your balance. (Hint: Engage your buttocks and abs for control.) Look straight ahead to find a focus point; it will help you establish balance and prevent you from leaning.

POSTERIOR DELTOID FLIES

Now we'll move on to the backs of the shoulders. This exercise helps to strengthen the rear of the shoulder girdle, which helps prevent slouching. It's also the muscle that helps you reach around to scratch your back.

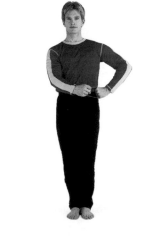

FIG. 1

Standing tall with your feet together, take the circleband in your left hand and make a fist around the band. Place your fist on your left hip. Reach with your right hand and grasp the other end of the band in front of you. Your left arm will remain folded at your hip. Extend your right arm in a diagonal across your torso, in front of your left hip. To start, your right hand will be positioned slightly out in front of your hip, but not touching it. The circleband shouldn't have any slack in it. Keep your spine long and erect. Look straight ahead.

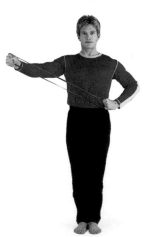

FIG. 2

Press your feet firmly into the floor and engage your legs, buttocks, and abs. Then lift your right hand out, up, and across your body, as if you're pulling a sheet off a bed or opening a door. Keep your arm straight and your elbow firm with a slight bend. Don't lock your elbow. Your elbow joint should point out to the side throughout the movement. Your palm should face into the center of your body. Lift your hand to shoulder height, hold, and release back to your left hip. Repeat. Exhale as you lift and inhale as you release.

Performance: Beginners—4 sets of 8 repetitions on each side
Advanced—6 sets of 12 repetitions on each side

Body logic: In this position you might tend to lean away or into the movement to gain leverage. To prevent this, spread your feet slightly until you have strengthened your core and found your balance. (Hint: Engage your buttocks and ab muscles for control.) Look straight ahead to find a focus point; it will help you find balance and prevent you from leaning.

SEATED ROWS

We'll now move to floor work and begin with our rowing circuit. Rowing, as you probably already know, is excellent exercise. It works your abdominals and lower back, which promotes good posture and a healthy spine. It also tones your arms and stretches your legs for positive mobility throughout the hip girdle.

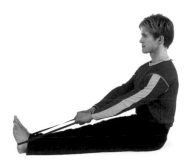

FIG. 1

Sit on the floor and extend your legs out in front of you, feet and knees together. Bend your legs and wrap the circleband around the arches of your feet. Hold the band in both hands between your second and third knuckles. Fully extend your legs out in front of you. Sit up tall through your spine and look straight ahead. Extend your arms straight out in front of you so your hands are navel height.

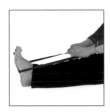

CLOSEUP DETAIL

Position the circleband around the arches of your feet. Press through the band with your feet. Keep your legs fully extended without locking your knees.

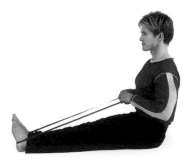

FIG. 2

Engage your abs and sit up tall from your sit bones through your head to support your lower back. Drop your shoulders down, and then pull your hands up to your chest, directly in front of your sternum. Hold, then release back down, bringing your hands to navel height. Repeat. Exhale as you pull and inhale as you release.

Performance: Beginners—4 sets of 10 repetitions
Advanced—6 sets of 15 repetitions

Body logic: In this position you might tend to lean back with the pull and lean forward with the release to gain leverage. To prevent this, sit up tall, engage your abdominals, and squeeze your buttocks muscles to support your torso.

LAWN MOWERS (CONCENTRATION ROWS)

Similar to Seated Rows, this exercise allows you to fully concentrate on the rowing movement, one arm at a time. Sometimes I like to refer to concentration exercises as those that allow you to feel how your body actually works. This understanding helps promote positive body control because you have to concentrate and focus intently on your movement, breath, and reaction to the movement. These types of exercises help you to better understand your body's language. Use concentration exercises to your full advantage, and learn what your body is capable of doing. In this exercise, we visualize pulling the rope starter on a lawn mower.

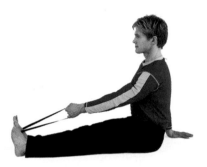

FIG. 1

Start seated upright with your legs extended, as you did for Seated Rows. Move the circleband to your right foot. Grasp the other end of the band with your left hand. Activate your feet, pressing through your heels, and keep your legs firm without locking your knees. Sit up tall through your spine and place your right hand directly behind you, in a stable yet comfortable position that allows your shoulder to remain in line with your waist and the floor. Keep your head level and look straight ahead at all times.

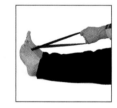

CLOSEUP DETAIL

Position the band around the arch of your foot. Activate your feet by reaching through your heels. Grasp the band between the second and third knuckles of your hand.

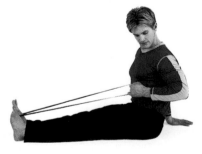

FIG. 2

Engage your abs and fully extend your left arm toward your right foot. Keep your hand at navel height. Exhale and pull your left arm directly back alongside your ribcage. Hold, inhale, and release. Repeat. Exhale as you pull and inhale as you release.

Performance: Beginners—4 sets of 10 repetitions on each side
Advanced—6 sets of 12 repetitions on each side

Body logic: In this position you might tend to lean back and to your side with each pull to gain leverage. To prevent this, sit up tall, engage your abdominals, and squeeze your buttocks muscles to support your torso. Push firmly with your supporting hand and keep your arm firm and stable. To gain better control of the movement, follow your hand with your eyes.

BACK/AB EXTENSIONS

This movement combines two exercises into one, strengthening your lower back and toning your abdominals. Both of these areas are important to maintaining a healthy spine and well-balanced posture. Remember, good posture helps your body function properly.

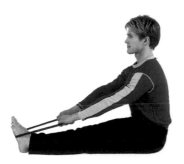

FIG. 1

Sit on the floor and extend your legs out in front of you, with your feet and knees together. Bend your legs and wrap the circleband around the arches of your feet. Hold the band in both hands between your second and third knuckles. Sit up tall through your spine and lean slightly forward until there is minimal tension in the circleband. Look straight ahead. Extend your arms straight out in front of you, keeping your hands at navel height.

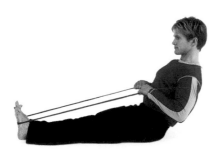

FIG. 2

Press firmly through your feet and activate your leg and buttocks muscles. Strongly engage your abs. Concentrate on your lower abdominals first—those below your navel. Pull your hands into your chest, directly in front of your sternum. Begin to slowly lean back, stretching the circleband, until you feel your abdominals fully engage from bottom to top. Hold and breathe. Use the band for support. Count to 3 and draw yourself up, using your abs to bring you to a seated position. Repeat.

Performance: Beginners—Work up to 6 repetitions, holding for 3 to 5 counts.
Advanced—Work up to 10 repetitions, holding for 5 to 8 counts.

Body logic: Pay attention to your body. Reach up tall through your spine throughout the movement. Keep your neck relaxed and look straight ahead. Maintain firm legs and reach through your feet. Only go back as far as is comfortable for you. You should be able to breathe comfortably while holding the extended position.

MODIFIED BRIDGE

Performing bridge exercises helps your body in many ways, including toning your quads and hamstrings and tightening your buttocks muscles. These exercises also help stabilize your hips and waist and help tone your abs. Including this exercise in your routine after performing abdominal exercises also helps to stretch the abs.

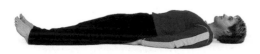

FIG. 1

Begin lying flat on your back with your feet hip-width apart. Stretch your body long and reach up through the top of your head. Place your hands at the sides of your buttocks for support.

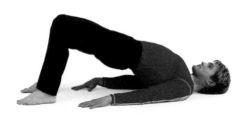

FIG. 2

Bend your knees, placing your feet flat on the floor. Move your hands out slightly wider than shoulder-width. Inhale, and as you exhale, squeeze your buttocks muscles, pressing your pelvic bone to the sky. Reach strong through your waist and elevate your hips to the bridge position. Breathe. Hold for a count of 3, then exhale and release. Repeat.

Performance: Beginners—Work up to 6 repetitions, holding for 3 to 5 counts.
Advanced—Work up to 10 repetitions, holding for 5 to 8 counts.

Body logic: Pay attention to your body. Keep your neck relaxed and look straight up. Don't overextend and compress your chest onto your neck. Maintain firm legs and press your feet firmly into the floor. Use your arms for balance and support. Raise your hips only as far as is comfortable for you. You should be able to breathe comfortably while holding your body in the raised position.

SIDE-LYING LEG RAISES

This exercise concentrates on toning and strengthening your hips and waist. This movement also helps promote mobility in your hips, waist, and pelvis—positively affecting your ability to walk, sit down, and stand up.

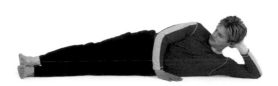

FIG. 1

Start by lying on your left side with your legs fully extended and stacked evenly on top of one another. Rest your head on your hand and elbow. Place your right hand directly in front of your abdomen at your navel. Your shoulder and upper arm should form a 90-degree angle. Keep your hips and waist level. Your hipbones should be stacked vertically, as should your shoulders and chest.

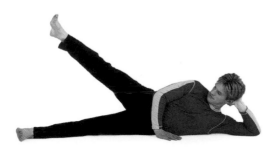

FIG. 2

Extend long through your left leg, engaging your abs. Press firmly into the floor with your right hand for support, reach out with your left elbow, and press down with your upper arm. Inhale; as you exhale, raise your right leg straight up from your hip to just above head height. Hold for a count of 2, inhale, and release back down. Repeat.

Performance: Beginners—Work up to 6 repetitions, holding for 2 to 5 counts, on each side. Advanced—Work up to 10 repetitions, holding for 5 to 8 counts, on each side.

Body logic: You might tend to roll your body forward and back. Keep your body stable by firmly engaging your abs. Don't overextend. Maintain a firm lower supporting leg and press firmly through your heel. Use your supporting arm to keep your body in the proper position. Make sure there's always even contact between your forearm and abdomen. Too much pressure means you're leaning forward. No pressure means you're leaning back. Only raise your leg as far as is comfortable for you without rolling your torso.

LEG RAISE AB CRUNCH

I call this exercise the concentration curl of abdominal work because it requires total focus on the abdominal muscles to get the maximum benefit. This exercise can give you a firm, flat stomach, which helps to support a healthy lower back and spine.

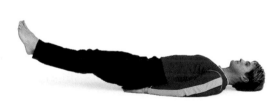

FIG. 1

Begin lying flat on your back, feet together and heels touching. Stretch your body long and reach up through the top of your head. Place your hands underneath the outside of your buttocks for support. You should feel your sit bones touching the insides of your index fingers.

FIG. 2

Inhale, and as you exhale, engage your lower abdominal muscles and lift your feet 6 to 8 inches off the floor. Engage your entire abdominal wall as you lift. Hold for a count of 3, exhale, and release slowly back to the floor. Repeat. Engaging the abdominal muscles from bottom to top is what provides the lifting action in this exercise. Don't lift your legs from your hips and waist; instead, use your abs to pull your legs up off the floor with minimal help from your hips. Press firmly down with your hands to help support the lift and release tension from your lower back.

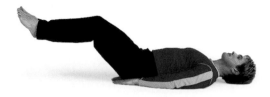

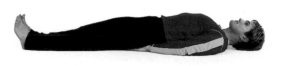

FIG. 3

If you're a beginner, start with your knees slightly bent and keep your knees bent throughout the exercise.

Performance: Beginners—Work up to 6 repetitions, holding for 3 to 5 counts.
Advanced—Work up to 10 repetitions, holding for 5 to 8 counts.

Body logic: Pay attention to your body. Don't arch your back and force leverage with your buttocks. Keep your neck relaxed and look straight up. Don't overlift and compress your lower back. Use your hands to support your buttocks and help keep your back stable. Maintain firm legs and reach through your heels. Use your arms for balance. Only raise your legs as high as is comfortable for you.

AB CRUNCHES

This is the classic belly-beautiful exercise. You can perform this exercise anywhere, anytime. Practicing this exercise throughout the day not only helps relieve stress but also helps to calm the body and draw positive focus to your breathing. Plus, toning and strengthening your abs helps to support your lower back and promote healthy posture.

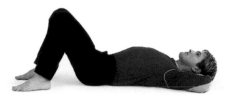

FIG. 1

Begin lying flat on your back with your knees bent and feet flat on the floor, hip-width apart, at a comfortable distance from your buttocks. Clasp your hands behind your head at the base of your skull. Keep your neck long and relaxed.

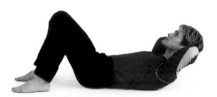

FIG. 2

Inhale, and as you exhale, engage your lower abdominals while lifting your head and upper shoulders off the floor. This is the starting and finishing position for this exercise. Press firmly and evenly through your feet, with equal pressure on the heel, ball, and toes of your foot. Keep your back flat and your buttocks engaged. Be sure your head is resting in your hands and not lurching forward to pull your shoulders up.

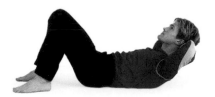

FIG. 3

Finish the movement by exhaling and engaging your upper abdominals, pulling your shoulder blades off the floor. Once you feel your shoulder blades rise off the floor, stop. Don't go higher. Hold for a count of 3 and release back to the starting position (shown in Fig. 2), with your upper shoulders off the floor and your lower abdominals still engaged. Inhale and repeat.

Performance: Beginners—Work up to 8 repetitions, holding for 3 counts.
Advanced—Work up to 12 repetitions, holding for 5 counts.

Body logic: Pay attention to your breathing. Use your breath to assist you in engaging your abs and reaching and lifting your shoulder blades off the floor. Don't arch your back and force leverage with your buttocks. Keep your neck relaxed and resting in your hands; look straight up. Don't jerk or force the lift and compress your lower back or strain your neck. Maintain firm legs and a long spine. Think "control"; don't force things. If you aren't strong enough to hold the lift at the starting point, then begin lying flat and work your lower abs. Lift your upper shoulders off the floor by engaging only your lower abs, then concentrate on engaging the entire abdominal wall. Slowly work to raise your shoulders and hold the starting position.

5

Balancing Your Diet

Do you live to eat, or do you eat to live?

If your diet is out of balance, chances are it's having a direct impact on your body's physiology and the state of your life. You're too tired to maintain your fast pace but you don't know how to slow down, so you reach for things to keep you going even though you're exhausted. It's no coincidence that you reach for stimulating, caffeinated, high-sugar, empty-calorie foods— the last thing your body needs—when you're most tired. You might try to wake up in the morning with some coffee, for example. Or maybe you drink several cups to keep you going throughout the day. Then later in the afternoon, when your head's about to hit the keyboard, you reach for a candy bar or a bag of cookies. Though what you choose to eat is ultimately under your control, the reflex that drives you toward these foods is not your fault. You crave sugary carbohydrates when serotonin levels get low. When that happens, you reach for empty calorie foods that don't do anything to nurture or support you and further throw your body off balance.

If you're tired and stressed, balancing the hormones that help center and calm you can be a challenge. The stimulating, high-sugar foods you eat to compensate for fatigue impact your body chemistry to further disrupt the balance of key components such as cortisol, serotonin, and melatonin. To make matters worse, your digestive system may shut down during stressful periods, so sometimes you simply lose your appetite altogether, skipping meals and paving the way for a blood sugar nightmare that's destructive to sleep and overall health. These patterns couldn't be worse for helping you get your rest.

Fast Food Isn't Good Food

Another destructive habit that's not conducive to a good night's sleep is eating fast food. With so many ways to process, refine, freeze, modify, or can food, we have transformed the way we eat in this country. Decades ago, when the fast food frenzy began, nutrition took a backseat to convenience, and rates for diabetes, heart disease, and cancer began to climb. We've been encouraged to believe that fast food is a lifesaver of some kind, that without it we'd be chained to our stoves and sinks in an endless cycle of stirring, washing, and drying. But it's possible to steam a delicious meal of fish and fresh vegetables in about the same 6 minutes it would take to defrost something in the microwave or wait in line at the drive-through. There are simple things you can do with broccoli, a nice lean piece of protein, and a wok that take half the time that it takes to pick up takeout.

Many of us can't understand why we have high cholesterol, diabetes, low energy, bad skin, and a weight problem when our older relatives lived into their 90s while smoking cigarettes, drinking coffee in the morning and whiskey at night, and eating bacon, eggs, and steak every day. But we need to ask ourselves, "How were they living?" Chances are they were active for most of the day, instead of sitting in front of a computer for hours at a time. They were probably eating food that wasn't heavily treated with pesticides, genetically modified, or stripped of its nutrients. They definitely weren't eating bags of fast food fries, hamburgers, pizza, or snack cakes. Food wasn't always such an "issue," either. Those relatives lived during a time when meals were ritualized and rest was an important part of every day. Foods were less processed, life was less stressful—and that made all the difference in the world.

Turning Off the Sugar Alarm

In our fast food haste, we've become a nation of unintentional gluttons. We eat too much because no matter how much we eat, we're still hungry. Our spirits are still hungry. This hunger for something more causes us to reach for unnecessary items at the grocery store rather than pausing to ask what it is that our bodies really need. Weight isn't the only concern when you're eating a convenience-food diet. Sugary and starchy foods are our tickets to a blood-sugar roller coaster, causing a spike and an inevitable drop in blood sugar. The brain lives on glucose. When blood sugar dips on top of the existing hunger, a hypoglycemia alarm goes off, putting the body in survival mode. The brain sends out signals saying, "Get me the quickest, most refined sugar you can find. No time to cook or break down brown rice. I need sugar, and I need it now!" The body translates this message to mean, "Must eat sweets," and goes for a cookie or a cola, which does nothing to provide a sustainable, slow supply of glucose. This causes another spike and dip in blood sugar, and the cycle continues.

However, it *is* possible to get out of the candy bar/soda pop loop. You can train your body to desire foods that help build a healthy hormonal balance and sustain blood sugar levels. Before your low blood sugar alarm normally goes off and you reach for sweets, soda, or even juice, make a conscious practice of eating a handful of almonds or other nuts, or nut butter on a celery stick or whole-grain bread. Not only will these healthy alternatives give your brain a steady source of glucose, but they will also aid assimilation of tryptophan, another essential component for a good night's sleep.

INSTILLING HEALTHY HABITS

Sometimes the best way to get out of an unhealthy cycle is to step back and take a look at your habits. Intention and awareness do a great deal to instill healthy habits. When you walk into a grocery store, what is your intention? When you sit down to a meal or go to grab a snack, do you have purpose? Ask yourself, what are you eating, and why? If you're just looking to fill your belly, you can expect almost anything in terms of the outcome. If your intention is to nurture and create balance, you'll be on your way to consistent, genuinely restorative sleep.

As soon as you realize how good certain foods make you feel, you'll instinctively make changes for the better. Look at what you eat and how it affects you. Do you know what you're eating? Keep a food journal and include how you feel before and after each meal or snack. Can you identify the food you put in your mouth? Do you eat foods that you know are good for you? How do you feel after a meal? Do certain foods affect you in specific ways, negatively or positively? Do you

ONE DAY AT A TIME

You don't have to give up all your unhealthy eating habits at once—just take things one day at a time. Gradually cut back on the stuff below, and remember, don't skip meals. That will just wreak havoc on your blood sugar.

✻ **Caffeine.** This stimulant is found in coffee, tea, soft drinks, and chocolate. Even one serving of caffeine in the morning is enough to disrupt your sleep at night. Try a week without it, and see if you're more able to answer your body's need for sleep.

✻ **Simple carbohydrates.** These include alcohol, sweets, and other foods containing refined sugars: pancakes, muffins, cakes, and breads made from white flour; white pasta; and white rice. Hypoglycemia, which is brought on by eating refined sugars, is directly linked to an inability to sleep.

✻ **Soda.** Not only is soda loaded with sugar and caffeine, but it also increases your risk of osteoporosis. In addition, low magnesium levels can account for foot and leg cramps.

✻ **Convenience foods.** Generally speaking, if the list of ingredients on the package contains words you wouldn't be able to recall in a game of Scrabble or words you've never even heard before, you don't want to put this food in your mouth. Natural ingredients are usually familiar, easy to pronounce, and wouldn't be your downfall in a spelling bee.

suffer from anxiety, indigestion, or gas after a meal? Or does eating make you feel clear, awake, and refreshed? Take note of the foods that just don't sit well with you, and see how you feel if you eliminate them from your diet.

Look at *how* you eat, and how it affects you. Do you eat at consistent times throughout the day? Do you eat off a plate, at a table, with silverware? Do you eat in front of the television, or while driving or walking? Do you simultaneously work, stress out, and have lunch?

You're not alone if you have days when, before you know it, one bonbon snowballs into an entire box, one piece of pizza turns into an entire pie, and so on. When this happens to you, take a look at what influenced your downfall. Are you more likely to binge on sugar when you haven't exercised or on days when you have a heavy workload? Is there a person or an event connected to those excesses? Do you see any pattern? Work to identify what's triggering your binging, and then become proactive in your efforts to change your eating habits.

EATING PROACTIVELY

The nutritional plan in this book is not intended as a sleep-improvement diet, though it can vastly improve the quality of your rest. It's more a way of life that will help promote physiological harmony, psychological peace, a happy spirit, an ideal body weight, optimum body function, a strong immune system, beautiful skin, *and* a good night's sleep.

Eating with intention, building a diet around foods that will fortify a healthy stress response and nourish your body's instinct for sleep, and keeping mealtimes sacred will do more than cushion your chemistry for sleep and stress management. It can cement your sense of control over your life. By eating proactively, engaging in conscious movement, and maintaining a positive frame of mind, you will face the world prepared. That's empowering.

In ancient Greek, diet, or *dieta,* means "way of life." Our food choices and the way we eat should complement the way we live. If you want to live a rich, focused, substantial, balanced, and peaceful life, your way with food should reflect those qualities. The whole-foods approach is the best diet for a holistic lifestyle.

Just as we're trying to get your system back in line with the rhythms of nature, a whole-foods diet will put you in contact with a more wholesome foundation. A whole-foods diet is based on eating local, seasonal, organic foods. If you eat this way, you'll avoid consuming chemicals, preservatives, pesticides, and refined products loaded with simple sugars. A whole-foods diet uses food for fuel, not for addiction. Fruits, vegetables, free-range meats, and organic cheese can be a wonderful expression of abundance. The whole-foods experience is mindful, plentiful, and focused on flavor, quality, and substance.

Eating in a way that is more aligned with nature allows our circadian rhythms to normalize. Circadian rhythms, which regulate sleep, are governed by light and oscillate with the seasons. These rhythms also rule appetite. Fine-tuning your circadian rhythms by eating a whole-foods diet can help reduce your sugar cravings. In time, you'll instinctively want the right foods at the right time.

Sleep Essentials

Following a whole-foods diet helps ensure that your body gets the nutrients it needs—including magnesium, calcium, and tryptophan—to maintain balance.

Magnesium and calcium are essential for nourishing the chemistry that helps us sleep deeply. Magnesium, a key nutrient that gets hit when we're under stress, is a very important balancer. Low magnesium is associated with the inability to stay asleep or sleep deeply, anxiety, constipation, fatigue, high blood pressure, irritability, and muscle cramping. Magnesium-rich foods include:

Amaranth, ½ cup	260 mg
Sunflower seed kernels, ½ cup	255 mg
Quinoa, ½ cup	179 mg
Spinach, 1 cup	156 mg
Wild rice, ½ cup	142 mg
Tofu, 4 ounces	118 mg
Halibut, 3 ounces	92 mg
Almonds, 1 ounce	86 mg

Brown rice, cooked, 1 cup	86 mg
Artichoke, 1 medium	72 mg
White beans, canned, ½ cup	67 mg
Millet, cooked, ½ cup	53 mg
Avocado, ½ medium	51 mg
Plantains, cooked, 1 cup	49 mg
Chocolate chips, ¼ cup	48 mg

Calcium is the most abundant mineral in the body. In addition to maintaining strong bones and teeth, calcium is important to much of the body's enzyme activity. If you have a calcium deficiency, you may suffer from muscle cramps, nervousness, hypertension, or insomnia. Calcium-rich foods include:

Mozzarella cheese, 3 ounces	621 mg
Sardines, canned with bones, 3 ounces	372 mg
Yogurt, plain, fat free, 1 cup	345 mg
Ricotta cheese, part skim, ½ cup	337 mg
Milk, fat free, 1 cup	302 mg
Orange juice, fortified, 1 cup	300 mg
Swiss cheese, 1 ounce	272 mg
Fortified cereal, 1 cup	250 mg
Oatmeal, instant fortified, cooked, 1 cup	215 mg
Salmon, canned with bones, 3 ounces	205 mg
Turnip greens, cooked, 1 cup	118 mg
Cheddar cheese, low fat, 1 ounce	118 mg
White beans, canned, ½ cup	96 mg
Broccoli, cooked, 1 cup	72 mg

Tryptophan is a major component in chemical balance and an essential building block for serotonin. It's the least abundant of the amino acids. Tryptophan deficiency contributes to insomnia. Inadequate amounts of tryptophan in the body have also been linked to depression, mania, and even to suicidal thoughts.

If you're on a high protein diet and find it difficult to stay asleep, consider adding some brown rice or other complex carbohydrates to your meals. Tryptophan is best assimilated when eaten in conjunction with a complex carbohydrate. The human body needs 80 to 250 milligrams per day. Combining tryptophan with vitamin B_6 and magnesium also enhances its effect. Foods rich in tryptophan include:

Cottage cheese, 1 cup	400 mg
Beef, 3 ounces	334 mg
Liver, 3 ounces	334 mg
Peanuts, 3 ounces	291 mg
Turkey, 3 ounces	283 mg
Tuna fish, ½ can	275 mg
Salmon, 3 ounces	231 mg
Halibut, 3 ounces	214 mg
Shrimp, 3 ounces	210 mg
Oatmeal, 1 cup	200 mg
Avocado, 1 medium	200 mg
Wheat germ, ¼ cup	110 mg
Egg, 1 medium	100 mg

In addition to consuming these nutrients, drinking enough water will also help you get to sleep. Inadequate sleep can lead to dehydration because your kidneys work harder and use more water to clean the body of toxins when you're tired. Give them a much-needed boost by keeping a full glass or bottle of water at your workstation, in your bag, and in your car.

Finally, maintaining healthy blood sugar levels is also essential to getting your Zzzs. Your brain lives on glucose, and when blood sugar dips, an alarm goes off in your body asking for fuel. If this happens in the middle of the night, it will wake you up.

STOCKING UP

Keeping your kitchen stocked with the following foods helps ensure that you'll always have ingredients for meals and snacks that will cushion your body chemistry for a good night's sleep.

* Agave sweetener
  (available at most natural food stores)

* Almonds

* Raw almond butter

* Apples

* Arame seaweed

* Bananas

* Berry jam

* Fresh or frozen blueberries

* Broccoli

* Cabbage

* Carrots

* Cashews

* Celery

* Cottage cheese

* String cheese

* Free-range chicken

* Cinnamon

* Eggs

* Flaxseed

* Frozen yogurt

* Low-fat goat's milk

* Grapefruit

* Halibut

* Hazelnuts

* Kale

* Lemons

* Lentils

* Mixed greens

* Oats

* Olive oil

* Oranges

* Pumpkin seeds

* Salmon

* Shiitake mushrooms

* Low-fat soy milk

* Strawberries

* Tofu (firm)

* Ground turkey

* Whole-grain bread

* Whole-wheat pastry flour

* White or brown Basmati rice

* Yogurt

Abstain from drinking juice or eating high-sugar foods, even fruits and sorbets, before bed; keep consumption of these things to a minimum during the day. Stick with complex carbohydrates and light protein, which burn slowly in the body, providing a consistent blood sugar level to feed your brain and body all day—and night.

THE 7-DAY SLEEP-WELL MEAL PLAN

The meal plan that you'll find on these pages is one that will nurture your body as well as your spirit. By using it as a springboard for changing your eating habits, you'll be setting yourself up for a lifetime of well-being.

DAY 1

BREAKFAST: Frittata with shiitake mushrooms and spinach or chard
(a healthy balance of protein and vegetables for a solid start to the day)

SNACK: ½ cup cottage cheese, ¼ cup almonds
(calcium, tryptophan, essential fats)

LUNCH: Whole-grain pita with avocado, sliced turkey, onion, and tomato
(magnesium, tryptophan, lycopene)

DINNER: Marinated seared tofu with brown rice and steamed vegetables
(calcium, magnesium, tryptophan)

DESSERT: Raw Bar; see page 137 (essential fats, fiber, magnesium, calcium)

DAY 2

BREAKFAST: Turkey, soy, or chicken sausage (2 pieces) with 1 whole-grain pancake
(hearty start to the day with protein, tryptophan, fiber)

SNACK: 1 cup cherries (fiber, melatonin)

LUNCH: Tuna and Brown Rice Salad; see page 122
(essential fats, fiber, balanced protein)

DINNER: Whole-grain fettuccine alfredo with grilled chicken and greens
(tryptophan, fiber, a balanced protein-to-carb ratio)

DESSERT: Blueberry Muffin; see page 138 (antioxidants, soluble fiber, potassium)

DAY 3

BREAKFAST: Whole-grain toast with eggs and broccoli
(fiber, antioxidants, protein balance)

SNACK: Super Nut Balls; see page 136 (tryptophan, essential fats, fiber)

LUNCH: Rice and Bean Salad; see page 118 (magnesium, calcium, fiber)

DINNER: Grilled yellowfin tuna with baked potato and kale
(essential fats, starch, fiber)

DESSERT: Strawberry Tart; see page 133 (fiber, vitamin C)

DAY 4

BREAKFAST: Tofu Scramble with vegetables and Banana Flax Bread; see pages 130 and 132 (phytonutrients, tryptophan, fiber)

SNACK: 1 orange, Cabbage and Apple Salad; see page 113 (antioxidants, fiber)

LUNCH: Caesar Salad with grilled chicken or fish; see page 116 (tryptophan)

DINNER: Baked Turkey Roll-Ups with rice and Swiss chard; see page 104 (tryptophan, fiber)

DESSERT: 1 cup plain yogurt with ½ cup berries (calcium and antioxidants)

DAY 5

BREAKFAST: Pineapple-Orange Smoothie with protein powder; see page 128 (antioxidants, protein, vitamin C)

SNACK: 1 protein snack bar, 2 rice cakes with 2 tablespoons hummus (fiber)

LUNCH: Whole-grain bread with sliced turkey, chicken salad, or egg salad; 2 carrots; 2 celery stalks (fiber, tryptophan)

DINNER: Chicken with brown basmati rice and broccoli (tryptophan, fiber)

DESSERT: Raw Bar; see page 137 (essential fats, fiber, magnesium, calcium)

DAY 6

BREAKFAST: Oatmeal with walnuts, cinnamon, and dried cherries (melatonin, fiber, essential fats)

SNACK: 2 fig bars, yogurt (calcium, fiber, tryptophan)

LUNCH: Mixed greens with grilled chicken and vinaigrette (tryptophan, protein)

DINNER: Vegetable Lasagna; see page 126 (fiber, protein, calcium)

DESSERT: Low-fat frozen yogurt with berries (calcium and antioxidants)

DAY 7

BREAKFAST: 2 scrambled eggs with whole-grain toast and ½ grapefruit (protein, fiber, vitamin C)

SNACK: ¼ cup raw almonds, 1 stick of string cheese (calcium, essential fats, fiber, protein)

LUNCH: Grilled Turkey Burger with mixed green salad and avocado; see page 105 (tryptophan, magnesium, essential fats)

DINNER: Grilled salmon with Kale and Seaweed Salad; see page 117 (essential fats, antioxidants, fiber, tryptophan)

DESSERT: Rice pudding with soy milk, cinnamon, agave, and cashews (vitamin B, folate, fiber, phytonutrients)

6

Recipes for a Good Night's Rest

Is your diet by design or by default?

A diet rich in legumes, whole-grain pastas and breads, and vegetables and fruits is designed to support a balanced, healthy lifestyle. Forming the foundation for that lifestyle are the nutrients represented in these recipes: lean protein, tryptophan, complex carbohydrates, and beneficial fats.

I've included protein sources that are high in tryptophan and low in saturated fats to help create a healthy hormone balance. These foods are combined with complex carbohydrates for ultimate tryptophan absorption. These meals are very nutrient dense and, from a carbohydrate standpoint, low on the glycemic index, which will keep blood-sugar levels steady. And they contain healthy, beneficial fats to support a decrease in inflammation and the well-being of the immune, cardiovascular, endocrine, and neurological systems. These healing fats also support psychological and emotional balance.

BAKED TURKEY ROLL-UPS

These protein-dense delicacies are great for lunch or dinner. Serve these tryptophan-rich turkey cutlets with calcium-rich greens and brown rice for a complete meal.

½	cup ricotta cheese
½	cup fresh spinach, chopped
¼	cup oats
2	tablespoons chopped fresh basil leaves
1½	pounds uncooked turkey breast slices, about ¼ inch thick
¼	teaspoon salt
¼	teaspoon pepper
½	cup chicken broth

Preheat the oven to 350°F. Spray a nonstick 9 × 9 × 2-inch baking pan with cooking spray. In a medium-size bowl, mix together the ricotta cheese, spinach, oats, and basil. Sprinkle each slice of turkey with salt and pepper.

Spread the spinach mixture evenly over the turkey slices; roll them up. Place the turkey rolls seam sides down in the pan. Pour the broth over the turkey rolls. Cover with aluminum foil and bake for about 25 minutes, or until the turkey is no longer pink in the center.

Serves 6.

Per serving: 166 calories; 4 g fat (25 percent calories from fat); 27 g protein; 3 g carbohydrates; trace of fiber; 74 mg cholesterol; 388 mg sodium

GRILLED TURKEY BURGERS

Turkey is a key building block for balance and calm. Enjoy these burgers on a whole-grain bun, over a bed of brown rice, or with a spinach salad with avocado and honey mustard dressing.

1	pound ground boneless, skinless turkey breast
¼	cup onion, finely chopped (about 1 small)
1	tablespoon tamari soy sauce
¼	teaspoon black pepper
1	tablespoon ketchup
2	tablespoons whole-wheat bread crumbs
2	tablespoons stoneground mustard
2	tablespoons horseradish

Preheat the grill. Mix together the turkey, onion, soy sauce, pepper, ketchup, and bread crumbs. Shape the mixture into 4 patties, each about ¾ inch thick. Grill the patties, turning once, until they're no longer pink in the center.

Mix together the mustard and horseradish, and spread the mixture on top of the burgers.

Serves 4.

Per serving: 181 calories; 3 g fat (16 percent calories from fat); 30 g protein; 7 g carbohydrates; 1 g fiber; 74 mg cholesterol; 500 mg sodium

TURKEY CUTLETS WITH CHERRY SAUCE

Turkey is one of the best dietary sources of tryptophan, an amino acid that the body converts into serotonin. Cherries contain fiber (pectin), vitamin C, and potassium, making this dish well rounded in nutrition *and* flavor.

1	tablespoon olive oil
1	teaspoon ground cinnamon
½	teaspoon black pepper
½	teaspoon salt
1½	pounds turkey breast tenderloins
⅔	cup apple juice
1	tablespoon arrowroot powder
1	tablespoon packed brown sugar
1	bag (16 ounces) frozen dark sweet cherries, partially thawed and drained

Heat the oven to 350°F. Spray a 13 × 9 × 2-inch rectangular pan with cooking spray. In a small bowl, combine the oil, cinnamon, pepper, and salt. Rub the tops of the tenderloins with the oil mixture. Place in the pan.

Bake uncovered for about 25 minutes or until the juice is no longer pink when the centers of the thickest pieces are cut.

While the turkey is baking, mix the apple juice, arrowroot powder, and brown sugar in a saucepan. Add the cherries to the saucepan. Heat to boiling, stirring constantly. Boil and stir for 1 minute; remove from heat. Cut the turkey into thin slices.

Serving suggestion: Serve the turkey over rice, and pour the sauce over the turkey.

Serves 6.

Per serving: 226 calories; 3 g fat (14 percent calories from fat); 25 g protein; 24 g carbohydrates; 2 g fiber; 61 mg cholesterol; 407 mg sodium

FETTUCCINE ALFREDO WITH CHICKEN AND BROCCOLI

This dish will satisfy your cravings for an evening starch. By using whole grain pastas, you'll increase your fiber intake without depriving your craving. The chicken balances the starch with beneficial protein, while the greens provide essential fiber, vitamins, and phytonutrients.

3	cups whole-grain fettuccine pasta
2	cups broccoli
1	cup 2 percent milk
½	cup chopped fresh parsley
½	cup grated low-sodium Parmesan cheese
4	ounces green onions, sliced (white parts only)
	White pepper, to taste
1	pound boneless, skinless chicken breast, grilled and chopped

Cook the pasta according to package directions in a 3-quart saucepan. Add the broccoli for the last 4 or 5 minutes of cooking. Drain and return to the saucepan.

In a large saucepan, bring the milk to a simmer over moderate heat. Stir in the parsley, cheese, and onions. Continue stirring until the cheese has melted and the sauce is thick and creamy. Pour over the cooked pasta and broccoli. Season to taste with white pepper. Stir in the chicken and cook over low heat for 4 to 6 minutes, stirring occasionally, until heated through.

Serving suggestion: Serve with a bed of mixed field greens.

Serves 4.

Per serving: 488 calories; 14 g fat (25 percent calories from fat); 40 g protein; 51 g carbohydrates; 5 g fiber; 129 mg cholesterol; 882 mg sodium

CHICKEN WITH SHIITAKE MUSHROOMS

Shiitake mushrooms offer immune support while chicken gives you an added boost of tryptophan. I love the flavor combination in this dish—and I hope you will, too!

1	tablespoon olive oil
6	skinless, boneless chicken breast halves (about 1½ pounds)
¾	pound shiitake mushrooms, coarsely chopped (about 5 cups)
1	medium leek, sliced (about 2 cups)
2	cloves garlic, finely chopped
2	tablespoons arrowroot powder
2	tablespoons water
2	cups chicken broth
½	cup dry white wine
1	teaspoon fresh oregano

Remove the fat from the chicken. Heat a large nonstick skillet over medium heat. Add the olive oil and chicken. Cook the chicken for about 12 minutes, turning once, until the juice is no longer pink when the centers of the thickest pieces are cut. Remove the chicken from the skillet and keep it warm.

Cook the mushrooms, leek, and garlic in the same skillet for about 3 minutes, stirring frequently, until the leek is tender. Mix the arrowroot powder with the water. Add this mix and the broth, wine, and oregano to the mushroom mixture. Heat to boiling, stirring occasionally. Boil and stir for about 1 minute, or until slightly thickened. Add chicken and heat through.

Serving suggestion: Serve over basmati rice or salad greens.

Serves 6.

Per serving: 217 calories, 5 g fat (20 percent of calories from fat); 31 g protein; 9 g carbohydrates; 2 g fiber; 68 mg cholesterol; 353 mg sodium

BROILED HALIBUT WITH SUN-DRIED TOMATOES

This light fish dish contains essential protein and lycopene-rich tomatoes. Halibut (which has a mild flavor) also supplies essential fats.

1	pound halibut fillets, about ¾ inch thick
8	sun-dried tomato halves (not oil-packed)
¼	cup olive oil
2	tablespoons chopped fresh parsley
1	tablespoon red onion, finely chopped

Preheat the broiler. Spray a thin coat of olive oil cooking spray on the broiler pan. Put the halibut on the rack in the broiler pan, about 4 inches from the heat. Broil for 7 or 8 minutes.

Place the tomato halves in 1 cup of hot water. Soak for about 5 minutes, or until soft. Drain and finely chop. Mix the tomatoes, olive oil, parsley, and red onion together. Spread over the top of the fish. Broil 1 or 2 minutes longer, or until the fish flakes with a fork.

Serves 4.

Per serving: 105 calories; 1 g fat (8 percent calories from fat); 21 g protein; 3 g carbohydrates; 1 g fiber; 49 mg cholesterol; 146 mg sodium

GRILLED SALMON SALAD WITH PEARS AND WALNUTS

Salmon is one of the best foods for supplying omega-3 fatty acids. When paired with fiber-rich pears and walnuts, this dish is off-the-charts delicious.

¼	cup olive oil
¼	cup balsamic vinegar
2	tablespoons lime juice
2	tablespoons honey
1	teaspoon salt
½	teaspoon pepper
4	salmon fillets
⅓	cup walnuts
4	cups greens
2	ripe Bartlett pears, thinly sliced

Whisk the olive oil, balsamic vinegar, lime juice, honey, salt, and pepper in a bowl until blended. Drizzle each fillet with 1½ teaspoons of the vinaigrette. Grill the salmon on an oiled, hot grill for 6 to 12 minutes per inch of thickness, turning once during cooking. Do not overcook.

To make the salad, spread the walnuts in a single layer on a baking sheet. Toast at 275°F for about 20 minutes, stirring occasionally. Toss the salad greens with some of the remaining vinaigrette, reserving some. Mound the salad greens on a large platter. Top with the pears, warm salmon, and walnuts. Drizzle the remaining vinaigrette over the salmon.

Serves 4.

Per serving: 481 calories; 26 g fat (47 percent calories from fat); 38 g protein; 27 g carbohydrates; 4 g fiber; 88 mg cholesterol; 662 mg sodium

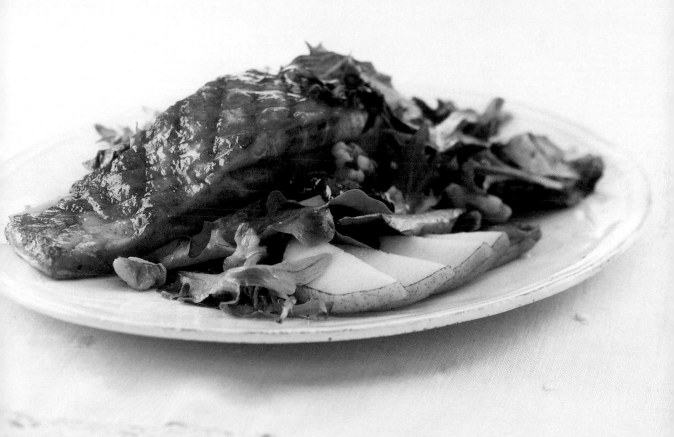

GRILLED SALMON SALAD WITH PEARS AND WALNUTS

LEMON-SHALLOT SCALLOPS

Seafood dishes don't get much easier than this one. You can enjoy these protein-rich scallops over whole-grain pasta, rice, or mixed greens for a dinner that is sure to satisfy your taste buds.

2	teaspoons olive oil
1½	pounds sea scallops
½	teaspoon sea salt
¼	teaspoon black pepper
2	teaspoons butter
3	tablespoons minced shallots
½	teaspoon minced garlic
¼	cup white wine
1	tablespoon fresh lemon juice
2	tablespoons finely chopped fresh parsley

Heat the oil in a large, nonstick skillet over medium-high heat. Sprinkle the sea scallops with the salt and pepper. Add the scallops to the skillet, and sauté for 2 minutes on each side. Remove the scallops, and keep them warm.

Melt the butter in the skillet. Add the shallots and garlic, and sauté for 30 seconds. Add the wine and lemon juice; cook for 1 minute. Return the scallops to the skillet, and toss to coat. Remove the skillet from the heat and sprinkle the scallops with parsley. Serve with lemon wedges, if desired.

Serves 4.

Per serving: 205 calories; 5 g fat (26 percent calories from fat); 29 g protein; 6 g carbohydrates; trace of fiber; 61 mg cholesterol; 531 mg sodium

CABBAGE AND APPLE SALAD

Both cabbage and apples provide cancer-fighting properties, as well as phytonutrients and fiber. This salad makes a terrific addition to a potluck lunch or dinner.

½   head red cabbage, shredded
4   whole carrots, shredded
1   Granny Smith apple, chopped
1½   teaspoons lime juice (fresh, if possible)
1½   teaspoons lemon juice (fresh, if possible)
        Salt, to taste
        Fresh cilantro, for garnish
        Fresh mint, for garnish

Mix the cabbage, carrots, and apple together. Transfer to a serving bowl and toss with the lime juice, lemon juice, and salt. Garnish with cilantro or fresh mint.

Serves 4.

Per serving: 49 calories; trace of fat (6 percent calories from fat); 2 g protein; 11 g carbohydrates; 3 g fiber; 0 mg cholesterol; 25 mg sodium

CURRIED CHICKEN HAZELNUT SALAD IN MELON SHELL

This summertime salad is full of healthy fats and antioxidants. Many of the herbs in curry (especially turmeric) act as natural anti-inflammatory agents.

2	cups cubed cooked chicken breast
½	cup diced celery
1	tablespoon finely chopped green onions
1	tablespoon capers, drained
⅔	cup chopped, dry-roasted hazelnuts
¼	cup low-fat mayonnaise
2	tablespoons plain low-fat yogurt
2	teaspoons curry powder
1	Granny Smith apple, cored and diced
	Lemon juice
3	cantaloupes or honeydew melons, cut in half, seeded, and drained upside down on a towel
	Currants, for garnish

Combine the cubed chicken, celery, onions, capers, and hazelnuts. Mix the mayonnaise, yogurt, and curry powder together, and stir into the chicken mixture. Cover and refrigerate for 4 hours or overnight.

To serve, add diced apples to the chicken mixture. Divide the mixture into 6 servings, and fill the cavities of the melons. Sprinkle currants over the top to garnish, if desired.

Serves 6

Per serving: 500 calories; 19 g fat (32 percent calories from fat); 24 g protein; 66 g carbohydrates; 6 g fiber; 57 mg cholesterol; 183 mg sodium

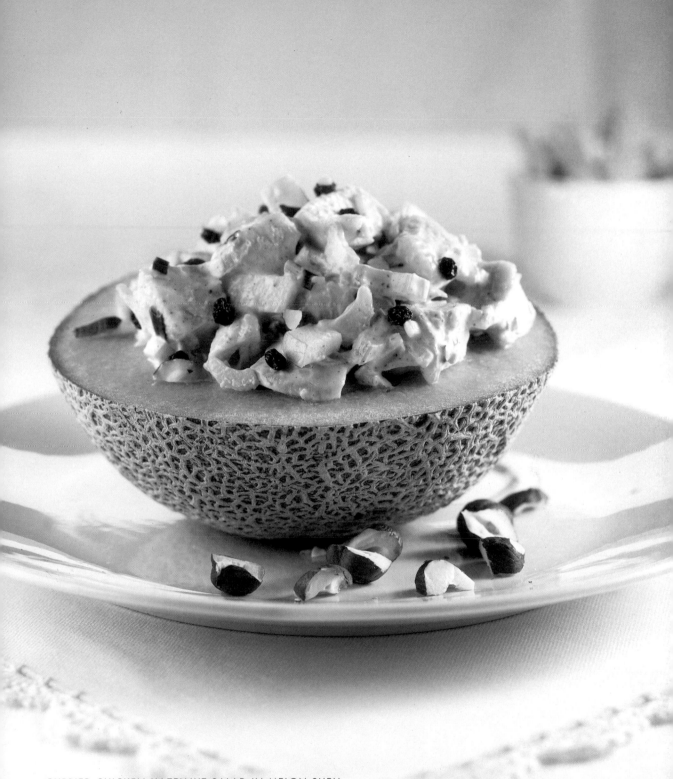

CURRIED CHICKEN HAZELNUT SALAD IN MELON SHELL

CAESAR SALAD

Here's a healthful makeover of a delicious classic. I like to serve this salad with a piece of grilled salmon or chicken, as well as a little bit of freshly grated Parmesan.

1	large bunch or 2 small bunches romaine lettuce
1	clove garlic
8	anchovy fillets
⅓	cup olive oil
3	tablespoons lemon juice
1	teaspoon low-sodium tamari soy sauce
¼	teaspoon sea salt
¼	teaspoon dry ground mustard
	Freshly ground pepper, to taste
⅓	cup grated Parmesan cheese

Remove any limp outer romaine leaves and discard them. Wash, rinse, and dry the remaining leaves (using a salad spinner or paper towels). Tear the leaves into bite-size pieces. You will need about 10 cups of romaine pieces.

Peel the garlic clove, and cut it in half. Rub the inside of the bowl (a wooden salad bowl works best) with the cut sides of the garlic. Allow a few small pieces of garlic to remain in the bowl, if desired.

Cut up the anchovies, and place them in the bowl. Add the olive oil, lemon juice, soy sauce, salt, mustard, and pepper. Mix well with a fork or wire whisk.

Add the romaine, and toss until well coated with the dressing. Sprinkle the Parmesan on top.

Serving suggestion: Add grilled chicken, fish, or tempeh to serve this salad as a complete meal.

Serves 5.

Per serving: 160 calories; 14 g fat (76 percent calories from fat); 6 g protein; 4 g carbohydrates; 2 g fiber; 8 mg cholesterol; 423 mg sodium

KALE AND SEAWEED SALAD

This salad makes a great side dish for lunch or dinner. The seaweed provides iodine, iron, potassium, calcium, and magnesium, while the kale supplies fiber, vitamin B_6, fiber, vitamin C, and potassium.

2	tablespoons olive oil
½	cup minced onion
½	cup arame seaweed, presoaked
1½	pounds kale or chard, trimmed and cut into 1-inch pieces
2	tablespoons toasted sesame seeds

Add olive oil and minced onion to a nonstick skillet and heat over medium-high heat. Drain the arame. Add the arame and kale, and stir-fry for about 5 minutes. Turn off the heat, add the toasted sesame seeds, and toss.

Serves 4.

Per serving: 130 calories; 9 g fat (60 percent calories from fat); 4 g protein; 10 g carbohydrates; 4 g dietary fiber; 0 mg cholesterol; 393 mg sodium

RICE AND BEAN SALAD

This salad contains vitamin B–rich rice and heart-healthy folate and potassium. You can easily prepare this recipe using leftover rice from a previous meal.

¼	cup cooked, long-grain brown rice
¼	cup cooked wild rice
½	red bell pepper, chopped
¼	cup white beans, cooked, rinsed, and drained
½	cup minced green onion
2	tablespoons chopped celery
2	tablespoons dried red or white currants
1	teaspoon lemon juice (fresh, if possible)
1	teaspoon olive oil
1	teaspoon crumbled blue cheese
	Salt and pepper

Combine the brown rice, wild rice, pepper, beans, onion, celery, and currants. In a separate bowl, whisk together the lemon juice and olive oil, and drizzle it over the salad mixture. Top with blue cheese. Add salt and pepper to taste.

Serves 1.

Per serving: 333 calories; 7 g fat (18 percent calories from fat); 11 g protein; 59 g carbohydrates; 8 g fiber; 2 mg cholesterol; 68 mg sodium

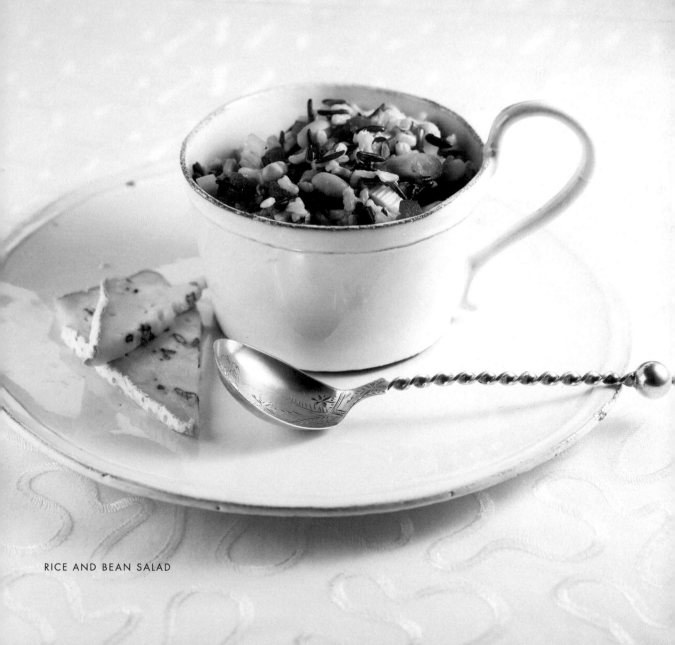

RICE AND BEAN SALAD

SCRAMBLED EGGS WITH SOUTHERN SALSA

This Southwestern-inspired dish is a great source of protein any time of day. And the phytochemical-rich salsa provides balance and helps promote disease prevention.

FOR THE SALSA:

½	red onion, quartered and sliced
½	yellow onion, quartered and sliced
2	jalapeño peppers, peeled, seeded, and chopped
2	cloves garlic, minced
5	tomatoes, peeled, seeded, and chopped
1¼	cups fresh cilantro
½	teaspoon chili powder
½	teaspoon freshly ground black pepper

FOR THE EGGS:

½	teaspoon garlic-flavored olive oil
4	eggs
2	teaspoons dried oregano
½	teaspoon onion flakes

To make the salsa, put the onions, peppers, and garlic in a blender or food processor. Coarsely mince. Add the tomatoes and cilantro; pulse gently until slightly chunky. Add the chili powder and pepper. Refrigerate.

To make the eggs, lightly coat a nonstick skillet with the olive oil. Heat over medium-high heat. Break the eggs in a mixing bowl. Add the oregano and onion flakes, and mix with a fork or whisk.

Pour the egg mixture into the skillet and scramble with a plastic spatula until cooked. Top with a few spoonfuls of Southern Salsa.

Serves 2. (*Note:* Salsa recipe makes 2 cups, so you will have leftovers.)

Per serving: 256 calories; 11 g fat (38 percent calories from fat); 15 g protein; 26 g carbohydrates; 7 g fiber; 374 mg cholesterol; 154 mg sodium

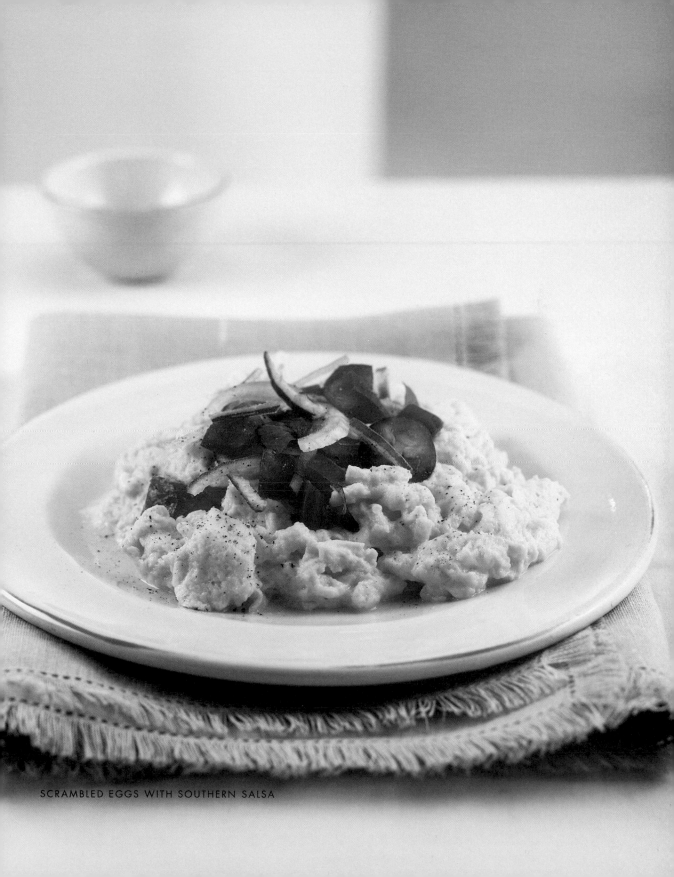

SCRAMBLED EGGS WITH SOUTHERN SALSA

TUNA AND BROWN RICE SALAD

Tryoptophan- and omega-3–rich tuna partnered with B vitamin–rich brown rice provide daytime balance and nighttime sleep. This meal is easy to prepare and travels well for a picnic lunch.

2½	cups cooked brown rice
1	can tuna in water, drained
1	hard-boiled egg, chopped
2	stalks celery, chopped
2	green onions, chopped
½	cup light mayonnaise
1	tablespoon fresh lemon juice
½	teaspoon Dijon mustard
	Salt and pepper

Combine the rice, tuna, egg, celery, and onions. Toss until mixed. Whisk together the mayonnaise, lemon juice, and mustard, and toss with the tuna and rice salad. Add salt and pepper to taste.

Serves 6.

Per serving: 274 calories; 8 g fat (27 percent calories from fat); 14 g protein; 35 g carbohydrates; 3 g fiber; 69 mg cholesterol; 321 mg sodium

LENTIL VEGETABLE STEW

Here's a satisfying stew rich in fiber and folate to warm your heart and soul. This stew is a thick and delicious vegetarian option for lunch or dinner.

2	tablespoons olive oil
1	cup chopped onion
½	cup chopped fresh parsley
2	cloves garlic, finely chopped
1	teaspoon ground cinnamon
½	teaspoon ground turmeric
½	teaspoon pepper
¼	teaspoon gingerroot, minced
3	cups water
2	cups chicken or vegetable broth
1	cup sliced carrots
½	cup (4 ounces) dried lentils, sorted and rinsed
1	cup brown rice, uncooked
1	can (15 ounces) whole tomatoes, undrained
¾	teaspoon sea salt
1	package (10 ounces) frozen green peas
1	package (9 ounces) frozen sliced green beans
3	sprigs mint, chopped
¾	cup plain, fat-free yogurt

Heat the olive oil in a Dutch oven or large skillet, and sauté the onion, parsley, garlic, cinnamon, turmeric, pepper, and gingerroot, stirring occasionally until the onion is tender. Stir in the water, broth, carrots, and lentils. Heat to boiling. Reduce heat, cover, and simmer for 25 minutes.

Stir in the rice, tomatoes, and salt, breaking up the tomatoes. Heat to boiling. Reduce heat, cover, and simmer for 20 minutes.

Stir in the peas, green beans, and mint. Heat to boiling. Reduce heat, cover, and simmer for about 5 minutes, or until the peas and beans are tender. Divide into 6 bowls, and garnish each bowl with a spoonful of yogurt.

Serves 6.

Per serving: 323 calories; 6 g fat (16 percent calories from fat); 15 g protein; 54 g carbohydrates; 11 g fiber; 1 mg cholesterol; 690 mg sodium

GINGERED CARROTS

The benefits of ginger coupled with carotene-rich carrots make this side dish not only a nutritional powerhouse but wonderfully tasty, as well.

3	cups sliced carrots
3	tablespoons maple syrup
2	tablespoons canola oil
½	teaspoon ground ginger

Heat 1 inch of water to boiling in a 3-quart saucepan. Add the carrots, and heat to boiling. Reduce heat to medium, cover, and simmer for about 5 minutes, or until the carrots are crisp-tender. Drain and set aside.

Heat the maple syrup, canola oil, and ginger in the same saucepan over medium heat, stirring constantly, until bubbly. Stir in the carrots. Cook for 2 to 4 minutes over low heat, stirring occasionally, until the carrots are glazed and hot.

Serves 6.

Per serving: 91 calories; 4 g fat (37 percent calories from fat); 1 g protein; 14 g carbohydrates; 2 g fiber; 0 mg cholesterol; 71 mg sodium

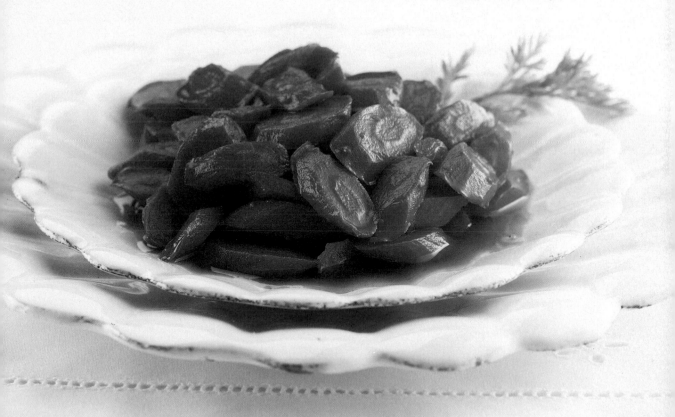

GINGERED CARROTS

VEGETABLE LASAGNA

This recipe offers the benefits of soy along with vitamin- and antioxidant-rich vegetables and pasta. Lasagna is wonderfully flexible, so have fun with this recipe. Play with the type and amount of vegetables you use. If you aren't a huge fan of bell peppers, for instance, use more broccoli or add some chopped spinach. Instead of part-skim mozzarella cheese, try substituting some goat's milk mozzarella. Experiment with whole-grain or rice lasagna noodles. And instead of chopping the vegetables in a food processor, chop them by hand, using that time to focus on your breathing.

1	package (16 ounces) lasagna noodles, uncooked
1	small container (15 ounces) part-skim ricotta cheese
1	cup mashed, firm tofu
1	egg
1	tablespoon extra virgin olive oil
2	cloves garlic, minced
1	small red bell pepper, thinly sliced
1	small green bell pepper, thinly sliced
1	cup thinly sliced onion
1	cup chopped broccoli
4	cups pasta sauce
1	tablespoon anise seed
1½	cups shredded part-skim mozzarella cheese

Cook the pasta according to package directions; drain. Lay the noodles flat on foil to cool.

Preheat the oven to 375°F. In a small bowl, stir together the ricotta, tofu, and egg.

In a medium nonstick skillet, heat the olive oil and sauté the garlic, peppers, onion, and broccoli for about 5 minutes.

Spread ½ cup of pasta sauce on the bottom of a 13 × 9 × 2-inch pan. Arrange 4 pasta pieces lengthwise over the sauce, overlapping the edges. Spread one-third of the ricotta mixture evenly over the pasta; spread 1⅓ cups of pasta sauce evenly over the ricotta. Sprinkle one-third of the anise seed over the sauce; spread one-quarter of the vegetables evenly over the sauce.

Repeat the layers two more times, ending with pasta. Spoon the remaining vegetables over the pasta and spread the remaining sauce evenly over the top. Sprinkle with mozzarella cheese. Cover with foil and bake for 50 minutes.

Remove the foil and bake for 10 minutes, or until hot and bubbly. Let stand for 10 minutes before serving.

Serves 8.

Per serving: 351 calories; 10 g fat (25 percent calories from fat); 19 g protein; 47 g carbohydrates; 3 g fiber; 39 mg cholesterol; 237 mg sodium

PINEAPPLE-ORANGE SMOOTHIE

Vitamin C-rich oranges combined with pineapple soothe and strengthen you for a busy day. By adding protein powder to this delicious smoothie, you ensure optimum blood sugar balance to help support you throughout your day.

1½	cups fresh pineapple chunks
½	cup orange juice
1	cup plain, nonfat yogurt
1	cup vanilla soy milk
2	tablespoons wheat germ
	Ice cubes, if desired
	Fresh mint, if desired
2	tablespoons protein powder, if desired (I recommend vanilla whey protein in this smoothie)

Place the pineapple, orange juice, yogurt, soy milk, wheat germ, ice cubes, and protein powder, if using, in a blender. Cover and blend on High for about 30 seconds, or until smooth. Garnish with the mint, if using.

Serves 3.

Per serving: 168 calories; 2 g fat (12 percent calories from fat); 4 g protein*; 35 g carbohydrates; 3 g fiber; 0 mg cholesterol; 13 mg sodium

*Note: Protein content will change if protein powder is added.

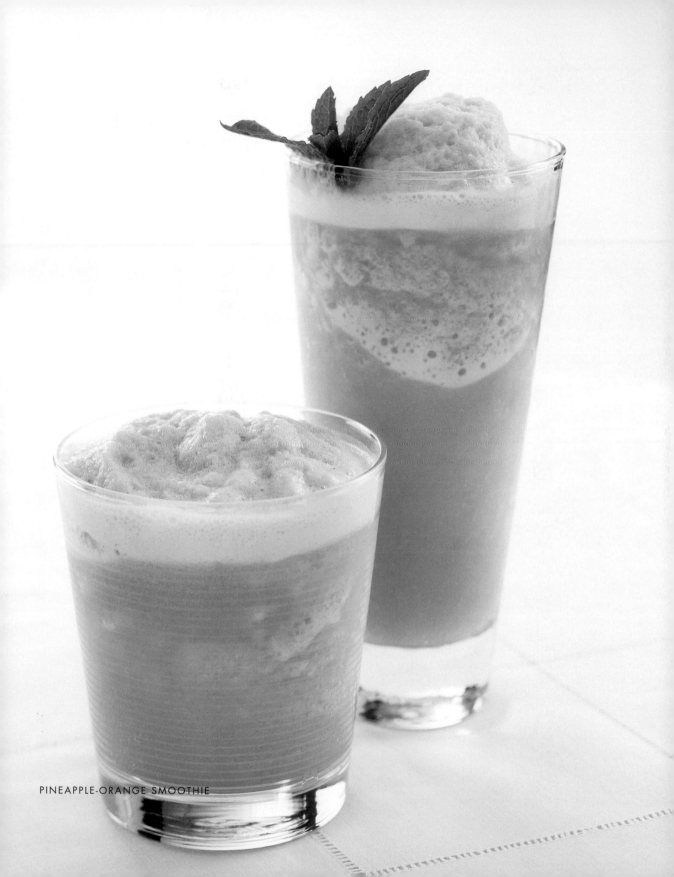

PINEAPPLE-ORANGE SMOOTHIE

TOFU SCRAMBLE

This is a "soysational" twist on a morning favorite—it's rich in heart-healthy soy. The tofu provides protein, magnesium, and calcium, while the spices add zing to this scrambled-egg alternative.

1	tablespoon olive oil
2	green onions, rinsed and chopped
1	carton (about 2 cups) firm tofu, mashed
½	teaspoon curry powder
½	teaspoon tamari soy sauce
½	teaspoon freshly ground pepper
1	carrot, chopped
½	cup broccoli
½	cup chopped zucchini

Heat the olive oil and green onions in a skillet over medium-high heat. Add the tofu and stir-fry for about 5 minutes. Add the curry powder, soy sauce, pepper, carrot, broccoli, and zucchini, and stir-fry for another 10 minutes.

Serves 4.

Per serving: 141 calories; 9 g fat (56 percent calories from fat); 11 g protein; 6 g carbohydrates; 3 g fiber; 0 mg cholesterol; 61 mg sodium

TEMPEH STIR-FRY

If you've been wondering how to use tempeh, this recipe couldn't be much easier. Tempeh is a great vegetarian food that packs phytonutrients and healthy protein. The vegetables add powerful antioxidant activity and round out this light meal that will satisfy most meat lovers.

2	tablespoons olive oil
12	ounces tempeh
1	clove garlic
1	teaspoon minced ginger
½	cup diced onion
1	cup chopped asparagus spears
1	cup rinsed and chopped kale
½	cup chopped zucchini
1	whole carrot, sliced
1	tablespoon tamari soy sauce
2	tablespoons water
	Other vegetables of choice

Heat the olive oil in a nonstick skillet or wok over medium-high heat. Sauté the tempeh, garlic, ginger, and onion for about 4 minutes. Add the remaining ingredients and stir-fry for about 10 minutes, or until the vegetables are cooked al dente.

Serves 4.

Per serving: 268 calories; 14 g fat (42 percent calories from fat); 19 g protein; 22 g carbohydrates; 2 g fiber; 0 mg cholesterol; 272 mg sodium

BANANA FLAX BREAD

Here's a whole-grain bread that provides beneficial fiber and fats along with potassium-rich bananas. This bread is great for breakfast or a quick snack—and it is something the whole family can enjoy.

½	cup brown sugar, packed
½	cup low-fat buttermilk (or soymilk)
2	eggs
3	tablespoons canola oil
¾	cup unbleached flour
½	cup whole-wheat flour
¾	cup ground flaxseed
1	teaspoon baking powder
1	teaspoon baking soda
⅛	teaspoon sea salt
1	cup very ripe, pureed bananas

Preheat the oven to 350°F. Coat an 8 × 4-inch loaf pan with nonstick spray.

In a large bowl, combine the brown sugar, buttermilk, eggs, and oil. Whisk until smooth.

In a medium bowl, combine the unbleached flour, whole-wheat four, flaxseed, baking powder, baking soda, and salt. Add to the liquid ingredients. Stir just until well blended. Fold in the bananas.

Pour the batter into the prepared loaf pan. Bake for 40 to 50 minutes, or until a knife inserted in the center comes out clean. Move the pan to a wire rack and let the bread cool slightly. While still slightly warm, turn the bread out of the pan and onto a wire rack, and let it cool completely.

Serves 10.

Per serving: 225 calories; 9 g fat (36 percent calories from fat); 6 g protein; 32 g carbohydrates; 5 g fiber; 38 mg cholesterol; 231 mg sodium

STRAWBERRY TART

This tart makes a great dessert or breakfast. The oats contribute fiber and melatonin while the berries provide antioxidants and fiber. If you're feeling especially indulgent, top your sliver of tart with some vanilla yogurt or frozen yogurt.

FOR THE CRUST:

⅔	cup rolled oats
½	cup unbleached flour
1	tablespoon sugar
1	teaspoon cinnamon
¼	teaspoon baking soda
2	tablespoons canola oil
2 or 3	tablespoons nonfat plain yogurt

Preheat the oven to 375°F. Coat a baking sheet with nonstick spray. Combine the oats, flour, sugar, cinnamon, and baking soda in medium-size bowl. Stir until well blended. Stir in the oil and 2 tablespoons of yogurt to make a soft, somewhat sticky dough. (Add the remaining yogurt if the dough is too stiff.)

Place the dough on the prepared baking sheet and pat it into a 10-inch circle. Place a 9-inch cake pan on the dough and trace around it with a sharp knife. Use your fingers to push up and pinch the dough around the outside of the circle to make a 9-inch circle with a rim ¼ inch high.

Bake for 15 minutes, or until firm and golden. Remove from the oven and set aside to cool. With a spatula, gently ease the crust onto a large, flat serving plate.

(continued on page 134)

FOR THE STRAWBERRY FILLING:

1½ pints strawberries

¼ cup all-fruit strawberry spread

½ teaspoon vanilla

Wash the strawberries and pat dry. Slice off the stems. In a small microwaveable bowl, combine the strawberry spread and vanilla. Microwave on high for 15 seconds, or until melted.

Drop a generous tablespoon of the spread on the crust and use the back of the spoon to spread it evenly over the crust. Arrange the strawberries, cut side down, over the layer of fruit spread. Brush or dab the remaining spread evenly over the strawberries, making sure that you get some of the spread between the strawberries to secure them.

Refrigerate for at least 30 minutes, or until the spread has jelled. Cut into wedges.

Serves 8.

Per serving: 117 calories; 4 g fat (29 percent of calories from fat); 4 g protein; 19 g carbohydrates; 2 g fiber; trace cholesterol; 43 mg sodium

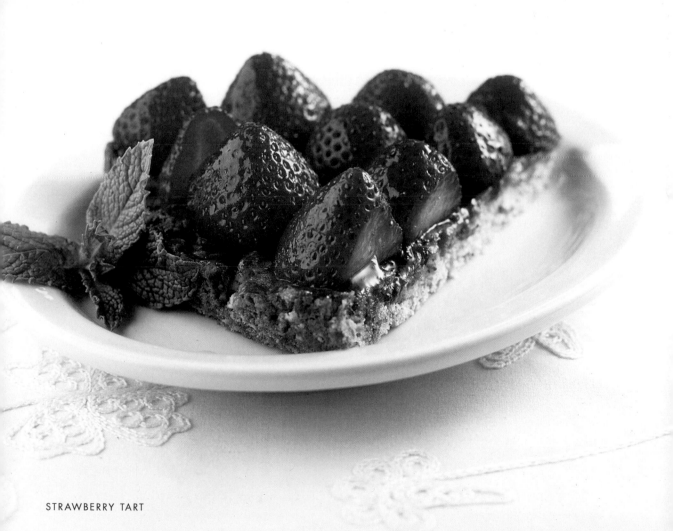

STRAWBERRY TART

SUPER NUT BALLS

You'll find that these nut balls are an energizing snack—one that's complete with minerals, fiber, and beneficial fats. Experiment with the recipe by adding your favorite nuts, seeds, or nut butters. Roll the balls in ground nuts; flaked, dried coconut, or carob or cocoa powder for a fun change.

⅓	cup ground almonds
⅓	cup ground pumpkin seeds, roasted
⅓	cup ground flaxseed
⅓	cup peanut butter
⅓	cup tahini
2	tablespoons maple syrup
	Dried, flaked coconut or chopped nuts
2	tablespoons protein powder (optional)

Mix all the ingredients together in a large bowl. The mixture should be somewhat tacky, but not "wet." If it seems too moist to work with, add more ground nuts. If desired, add protein powder for an extra burst of protein. Take about 1 tablespoon of the mixture and roll it into a ball, then roll it in dried coconut or chopped nuts. You can eat the balls right away or place them on a cookie sheet and refrigerate them for a firmer snack. Store leftover balls in an airtight container in the refrigerator.

Makes about 10 balls; each ball is 1 serving.

Per serving: 172 calories; 13 g fat (66 percent calories from fat); 6 g protein*; 10 g carbohydrates; 4 g fiber; 0 mg cholesterol; 52 mg sodium

* *Note:* Protein content will change if protein powder is added.

RAW BARS

Rich in minerals, fibers, and beneficial fats, these bars are energizing and satisfying. Definitely a Rouse-house favorite.

1½	cups dates, pitted
¼	cup ground flaxseed
½	cup almonds
½	cup cashews
½	cup walnuts

Soak the dates in water for a few hours or overnight. Drain them and process them in a food processor with the flaxseed, almonds, cashews, and walnuts. Blend until well mixed. Press the mixture into an 8 × 8 × 2-inch baking pan. Allow it to sit in the oven either with no heat or at 90°F for several hours. This will dehydrate the mixture somewhat and make it less sticky. Slice into bars.

Serves 8.

Per serving: 262 calories; 15 g fat (52 percent of calories from fat); 7 g protein; 31 g carbohydrates; 6 g fiber; 0 mg cholesterol; 5 mg sodium

BLUEBERRY MUFFINS

These muffins are full of antioxidant-rich blueberries and whole-grain goodness. Enjoy these at breakfast with a poached egg or yogurt—or have one for a snack at any time of day.

1	cup blueberries, fresh or frozen
1	cup low-fat or reduced-fat milk
¼	cup applesauce
½	teaspoon vanilla
2	tablespoons plain, nonfat yogurt
1	egg
2	cups whole-wheat flour
⅓	cup sugar
3	teaspoons baking powder
½	teaspoon salt

Preheat the oven to 400°F. Lightly coat the bottoms of 6 regular-size muffin cups with canola oil cooking spray, or line each cup with a paper baking cup.

Rinse the blueberries with cool water, and discard any crushed berries. Remove any stems.

Beat the milk, applesauce, vanilla, yogurt, and egg in a large bowl with a fork or wire whisk until well mixed. Stir in the flour, sugar, baking powder, and salt all at once, just until the flour is moistened. (The batter will be lumpy.)

Carefully fold in the blueberries.

Spoon the batter into the muffin cups, dividing the batter evenly.

Bake for 20 to 25 minutes or until golden brown. Immediately remove the muffins from the pan to a wire cooling rack. Serve warm or cool.

Makes 6 regular-size muffins.

Per serving: 101 calories; 2 g fat (14 percent calories from fat); 3 g protein; 20 g carbohydrates; 1 g fiber; 34 mg cholesterol; 456 mg sodium

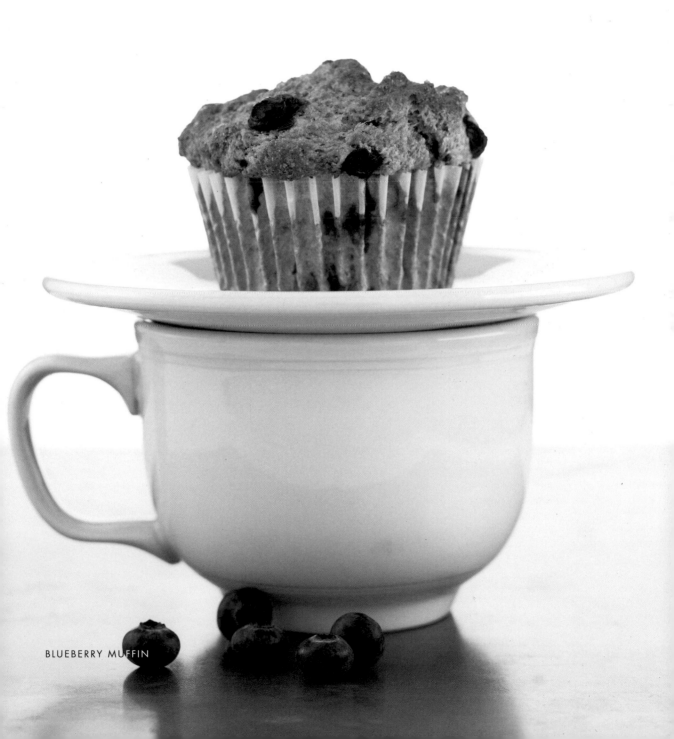

BLUEBERRY MUFFIN

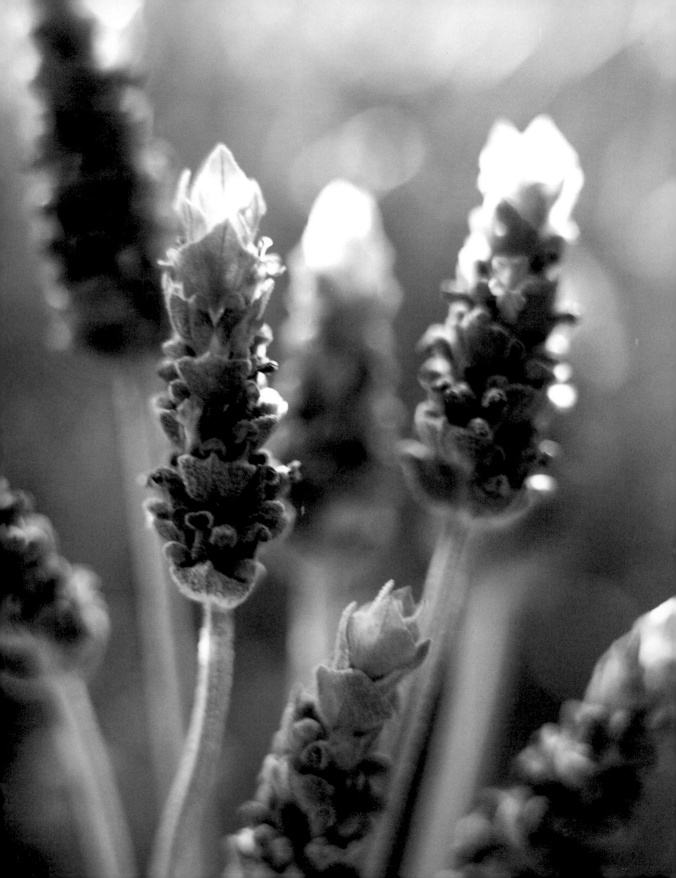

7

Short-Term Remedies

Is there more to life than merely increasing its speed?

Once you put into practice the advice I've offered in the previous chapters of this book, you should rarely have a restless night. But that's not to say you won't ever have a night where you have trouble sleeping. Every so often, you probably will.

That's where this chapter of the book comes in. Over the following pages I've detailed short-term solutions for getting back to sleep—quick fixes for the sleepless mind and body. Try all of them—or just your favorites—and you're guaranteed a deep, satisfying sleep.

Mending Your Mind

Your mind will let you rest as soon as you identify any thoughts that aren't supporting feelings of peace. Are you regretting something that happened in the past? Are you wishing for a different outcome to something that happened? If so, simply allow yourself to see the event as no longer relevant. It's over. Gone. Out of your life. Assure yourself that given another opportunity, you might choose differently. Bless the lesson and let it go.

If you're focusing on the future and feeling ambivalence, anxiety, excitement, or fear, allow yourself to bring your thinking back to the present. Confidently release that future moment and allow for peace in its place.

Breathe into any places of tension or unease. Breathe into the places of hurt with love and compassion. Open your heart to allow warm energy in, and allow it to wash over you with each breath. Allow your breath to dissolve any feelings of discontent. Let your breath roll over any doubt, fear, or feelings of guilt and judgment.

If you're holding any feelings of resentment toward another person, notice the feeling and again, open your heart. Allow only love to shine through.

Using Aromatherapy

The soothing scent of aromatherapy oils can help you relax and lull you back to sleep. Place the oils in a diffuser, sprinkle a few drops on your pillow, or rub a drop on your clavicle. Try basil, bergamot, chamomile, lavender, mandarin, marjoram, petit grain, rose, sandalwood, or ylang-ylang.

Note: Most essential oils should never be applied to your skin full-strength. Before applying, dilute them in an oil (almond oil works well), cream, or gel before application. Lavender and rose are exceptions and can be applied undiluted. Because essential oils can cause skin irritation or allergic reactions, always do a patch test before applying oil to your skin. To perform the patch test, put a few drops of the essential oil mixed with the carrier base on the back of your wrist. Then wait for an hour or more. If irritation or redness occurs on the area where you applied the oil, wash the area with cold water. Retest using half the amount

DO THE Bs TO HELP YOU GET YOUR Zzzzs

✳ **B**rew a cup of chamomile or lemon balm tea.

✳ Read a **B**ook that soothes and nourishes your heart and spirit.

✳ Draw a warm **B**ath to help support your ideal temperature for sleep (60° to 68°F), and add a few drops of lavender oil to the water. (See the opposite page for tips on using essential oils safely).

✳ Go to the **B**athroom to help you feel more comfortable and to avoid waking up at night.

✳ **B**e grateful. If you take a feeling of gratitude to sleep, you'll wake with an attitude to keep.

✳ **B**reathe in peace. Breathe out tension, mind chatter, and self-defeating thinking.

of oil. If you don't experience any irritation, just use half the amount on your skin. Of course, if your skin becomes irritated, avoid the oil entirely.

As an additional safety precaution, never apply essential oils to skin that's cut or abraded, and always keep essential oils away from your eyes. Avoid using essential oils if you're pregnant or nursing.

Munching a Midnight Snack

An empty stomach may wake you up in the middle of the night. To satisfy your belly, keep a snack on your nightstand. Good choices include an oatmeal cookie or a whole-grain granola bar. That way, if you wake up hungry, you'll have a snack right at your fingertips.

BODY WORK

Other short-term solutions for getting back to sleep involve helping your body—as opposed to your mind—relax. Here are some ways to do just that.

Self-Massage/Acupressure

The practice of acupressure is the oldest form of massage, having been developed many thousands of years ago. By asserting pressure with your fingers or hands on specific areas of the body, you release trapped energy that causes the ailment. Used consistently, acupressure can be an effective self-treatment for tension-related problems. Perform each movement for up to 2 minutes at a time, several times a day.

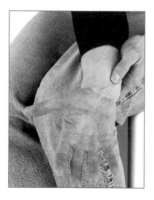

FIG. 1

To help clear and cleanse your mind, massage along the inside (medial aspect) of your wrist, from roughly 4 inches above your wrist joint (up the forearm) toward your wrist crease. You can use your thumb and gently "walk" it down this area of your forearm while you breathe, pressing gently as you go.

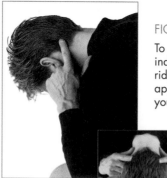

FIG. 2

To help relax and release stress, use your thumb or index finger to massage pressure along the occipital ridge at the base of your skull. Breathe slowly as you apply firm pressure with both hands on either side of your head, then release.

Reflexology

Reflexology defines specific areas on your hands and feet that correspond to every other part of your body. We can ease discomfort in the body and mind by stimulating the appropriate reflexology or reflex area. You can use reflexology to relieve stress and tension and to help stimulate deep relaxation. Practicing reflexology consistently helps to harmonize and balance the entire body. Perform each movement for up to 2 minutes at a time, several times a day.

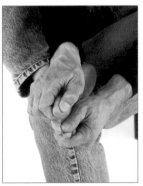

FIG. 1

To help release stress, massage the arches of your feet. This area corresponds with the adrenal glands. With your thumb, apply firm pressure along the inside arch area.

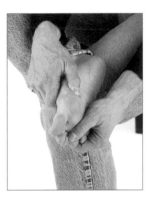

FIG. 2

You can also use reflexology on the area that corresponds with your pineal gland, which is responsible for releasing melatonin. Apply firm pressure to the ends of your big toes. Work along the bottom of the tip of each big toe as you breathe slowly and deeply.

YOGA

Many yoga postures can help alleviate specific health conditions, yet the best way to take full advantage of yoga is to begin simply and allow your own yoga practice to develop into a program that best suits your needs. Whether you're performing a simple sequence of poses or performing just one pose at a time, the benefits are endless. Use the following postures independently or in sequence to help balance your body and mind when you feel the need to release tension or stress. Perform each posture in the sequence shown, from start to finish. Hold each posture for 5 long, even breaths, and then move to the next posture.

MOUNTAIN POSE WITH ARMS OVERHEAD

The opening of this sequence is made up of two postures that establish the first part of the traditional Sun Salutation. Mountain Pose is the basic standing posture in yoga, which includes Mountain Pose with Arms Overhead. Positioning your body properly and concentrating on standing and reaching tall helps you find your body's proper alignment, reduce stiffness and tension caused by incorrect posture, and support your spine in its healthiest form.

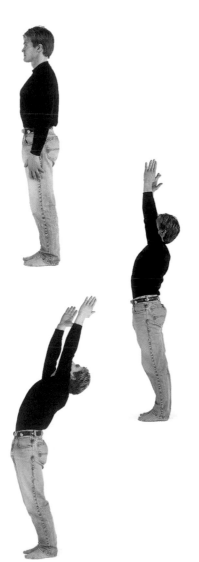

FIG. 1

Stand tall with your feet together and extend your arms down along your sides, fingers pointing toward the floor. Reach up tall through your head, looking straight ahead. Create a strong foundation with your legs, keeping your buttocks firm and stomach soft. Lift your chest, spine, and neck straight up, as if a rope is pulling you skyward through the center core of your body. Breathe. Breathe deeply and consistently.

FIG. 2

Inhale, and as you exhale, raise your arms overhead, hands shoulder-width apart, fingers reaching skyward. Reach as tall as you can. Do not hunch your shoulders or relax your neck. Keep your legs active, pressing through your feet, buttocks firm and stomach soft. Breathe deeply, reaching taller on each exhalation.

FIG. 3

As you establish a relaxed, extended pose, reaching as tall as you can with your arms, gradually lean your upper body back, bending from your waist and reaching up through your chest. Breathe. Hold for 2 or 3 long, comfortable breaths, and release back up to vertical.

STANDING FORWARD BEND (RAG-DOLL ASANA)

Forward Bend is one of the best postures for relieving stress and calming the nervous system. The posture helps to stretch the spine and backs of the legs and improves blood circulation to the upper body, head, and brain. This combined effect helps relieve tension in the spine and stress on the brain.

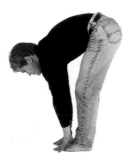

FIG. 1

From Mountain Pose with Arms Overhead, bend your knees slightly. Inhale, then exhale while bending forward from your waist, placing your hands on the floor alongside your toes. Keep your back straight and your neck soft. Keep your spine long and extended, allowing your legs to stretch easily. Breathe deeply into the areas that seem tight, extending and lengthening on each exhalation. Do not force your torso down, but allow it to hang freely from your hips.

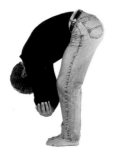

FIG. 2

Another variation of the Forward Bend is to cross your arms and hold your elbows, allowing your upper body to hang from your hips. This is called the Rag-Doll Asana and can be performed anytime, anywhere, when you feel the effects of stress or tension weighing you down.

MOUNTAIN POSE WITH ARMS OVERHEAD

You'll complete this short sequence with the starting posture: Mountain Pose. This allows you to find your center, focus your mind, and establish complete balance in your body.

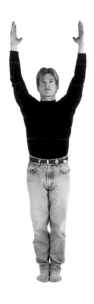

FIG. 1

From Forward Bend, inhale. On the exhalation, reach long through your arms and lead with your chest to raise your body back up to standing, reaching your arms overhead all in one motion. Concentrate on reaching tall and creating length through your hips and waist. Keep your legs firm. Reach as tall as you can. Breathe.

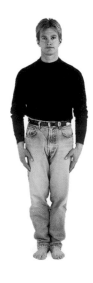

FIG. 2

Inhale deeply and on the exhalation, slowly lower your arms down alongside your body. Stand tall, releasing your shoulders down and away from your ears. Keep your legs firm and balanced evenly between the balls and heels of your feet. Stay here for a few minutes, taking long slow breaths to feel the grounding effect of this posture.

Repeat the sequence 3 to 5 times consecutively for maximum benefit and relief.

CHILD'S POSE

Child's Pose is a restorative posture that allows you to relieve pressure on your lower back, realign your spine, and relieve tension in your head and brain through the action of resting your forehead on the floor. This posture also helps develop proper abdominal breathing.

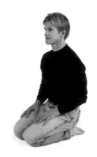

FIG. 1

Kneel on the floor with your knees and feet touching. Rest your buttocks back on your heels and sit up tall.

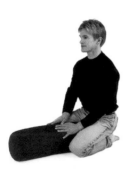

FIG. 2

Spread your knees just far enough apart to pull the bolster in between them. The bolster should rest about halfway up your thigh and your feet should still be touching each other. Sit upright and maintain a long spine.

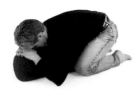

FIG. 3

Inhale deeply. As you exhale, slowly drop your torso forward. Rest your chest and forehead on the bolster. Reach your arms out and wrap them around the end of the bolster. Allow your entire body to rest comfortably on the bolster. Let your legs relax and spread open slightly, if necessary. You should feel the weight of your body resting on your thighs and tension releasing from your back. Take many long, deep breaths in this position. Continue to allow your body to fall into the bolster. Breathe.

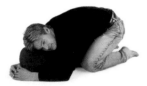

FIG. 4

Once you're comfortable and relaxed, exhale and turn your head to the left. Rest here for 10 long, deep, even breaths. Then turn your head to the right for 10 more breaths.

RESTORATIVE TWIST

This simple, restorative twist helps you relieve pressure and tension in your lower back. Allowing your upper body to rest comfortably on the bolster with your hips and waist suspended below your heart helps gently stretch and open your hips and waist with your body's own weight. This posture helps reverse the effects of standing and sitting throughout your day.

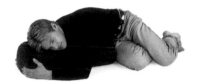

Slowly come up from Child's Pose and place the bolster against your hip. Then place your belly, chest, and the side of your face on the bolster. Allow your hips to twist and your upper leg to rest gently on your lower leg.

Slowly come up and change to other side, breathing into your hips as you allow them to open and fall into the ground below you.

Slowly come up to sitting on your sit bones. Move the bolster end to your sit bones and place your feet on top of the bolster. Let you knees fall to the side and open fully while keeping your feet together.

Place your hands gently on your belly. Let your breath fully rise and fall, releasing tension. Allow peace to envelop your body and mind.

RECLINED COBBLER

Reclining in this posture with your legs and feet raised above your heart and your knees opened out to the sides helps to stretch your inner thighs, hips, and waist. Increasing blood flow to the pelvic region assists in digestion, and the increased circulation to the head helps calm the flow of thoughts to relax your mind.

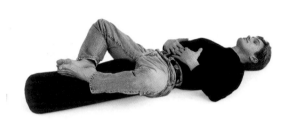

Move back up to a seated position with your legs extended out in front of you. Gently lie down and bend your knees with your feet flat on the floor. Pull the end of the bolster into your body, so it touches your buttocks. Place your feet up on the bolster and gently allow your knees to fall open toward the floor. Breathe into your hips, and allow the pose to open and relax your entire midsection. As you begin to relax, place your hands on your belly and feel the rise and fall of your abdomen. Listen to your breath and allow the movement of your breath to calm and relax you.

SAVASANA WITH BLANKET

The word *Savasana* means "corpse," and in this posture your body is completely still and motionless while your mind is focused and calm. This postures helps to relieve fatigue and achieve total relaxation. Begin by using a blanket across your abdomen, which helps to focus your mind on your breath and the rise and fall of your belly. This allows you to let go of all other thoughts.

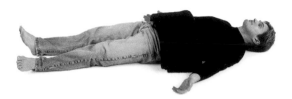

Lie flat on the floor and place a folded blanket across your belly. Spread your feet hip-width apart, and allow your legs to fall open. Relax your shoulders down and away from your neck. Extend your arms out slightly wider than shoulder width, palms facing up and hands open. Relax your head and close your eyes. Breathe deeply.

SAVASANA WITHOUT BLANKET

When you are more centered and able to find calm within your thoughts, move to the traditional posture, practiced without a blanket. This posture allows you to completely surrender, deepening your breath to slow your heart rate and increasing the flow of oxygen to every part of your body. Practice this pose before or after any physical activity or simply to release built-up tension and stress.

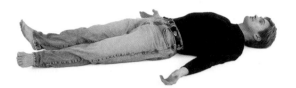

Lie flat on the floor. Spread your feet hip-width apart, and allow your legs to fall open. Relax your shoulders down and away from your neck. Extend your arms out slightly wider than shoulder width, palms facing up and hands open. Relax your head and close your eyes. Breathe deeply.

Index

Underscored page references indicate boxed text and tables. **Boldface** references indicate photographs.

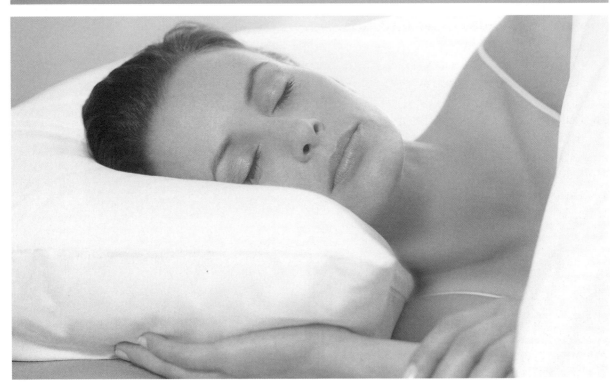

Sleep better tonight with *Health Solutions for Sleep*

Proven relief from sleeplessness is in your own hands — without side effects or habit-forming drugs

Get to sleep faster, sleep more soundly every night, and feel more rested and rejuvenated every morning! The advanced *Health Solutions for Sleep* programs and kits restore sound, healthy sleep cycles through simple yet powerful nutrition, relaxation techniques, insights on setting up your internal and external sleep environments, and other natural solutions.

- Gives you quick-relief checklists, recipes, guided relaxation techniques, and more
- Clinically proven, simple to use, and easy to customize to your lifestyle
- Guided by naturopathic physician, fitness expert, author, and chef Dr. James Rouse
- Naturally and effectively rebalances sleep-promoting biochemistry
- Reduces risk of insomnia-related illnesses including depression and chronic fatigue

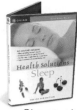

Health Solutions for Sleep DVD

The comprehensive program!
Lasting lifetime solutions plus practical
quick-relief remedies.

Give your body what it needs to treat the underlying causes of sleeplessness and foster healthy sleep cycles every night. Dr. James Rouse guides you through relaxation and breathing techniques, self-massage, and other quick-relief remedies for times when you're having trouble sleeping. Restorative yoga with renowned yoga master Rodney Yee helps balance energy levels so you can sleep at night and feel rejuvenated in the morning. Dr. James also gives you insight on creating a restful environment, plus foods and meal preparation tips that help rebalance natural sleep hormones. Also includes an in-depth guidebook with frequently asked questions, a checklist to help remedy sleeplessness when it strikes, a quick-reference list of sleep-supportive foods and nutrients, and a 7-day menu plan with recipes to help you incorporate sleep-friendly foods into your life. 1 hour 50 minutes.

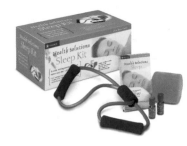

Health Solutions for Sleep Kit

Targeted A.M. and
P.M. tools and
techniques for fast,
effective relief from
sleeplessness!

Fall asleep quickly, stay asleep all night, and feel renewed and rejuvenated every morning with this practical kit. Dr. James Rouse shows you quick, easy-to-do evening tension-relief, self-massage, and restorative yoga techniques, plus an energizing morning resistance-cord workout to energize you and rebalance daytime and nighttime energy. Included workout and tension-relief tools, Sleep Blend aromatherapy oils and how-to guide with sample sleep-friendly recipe help you start sleeping better tonight. Includes aromatherapy tips plus an overview of how exercise can help you restore natural sleep patterns.

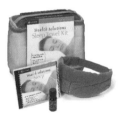

Health Solutions for Sleep Travel Kit

Lets you take effective
sleep-enhancing tools
anywhere you go!

Wherever you are, you can create a restful environment and enjoy deep, restorative sleep with this easy-to-carry kit. On audio CD, Dr. James Rouse guides you through a soothing relaxation and breathing sequence followed by gentle instrumental music to help lull you to sleep. Included are a soft, adjustable fleece-covered sleep mask and relaxing Sleep Travel Blend aromatherapy oil, plus a helpful travel-sleep guide with recipe for an on-the-go, sleep-promoting snack.

Also available:

Health Solutions for Stress Relief

- **Deluxe DVD** with comprehensive, lasting solutions for managing stress
- **A.M Stress Relief Kit** with stress-resilience boosting tools and workout to begin the day
- **P.M Stress Relief Kit** with calming evening tools and routine
- **Stress Relief Travel Kit** for keeping stress in check anywhere you go

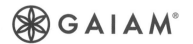

THE ART OF LIVING IN HARMONY

with

YOURSELF AND YOUR WORLD

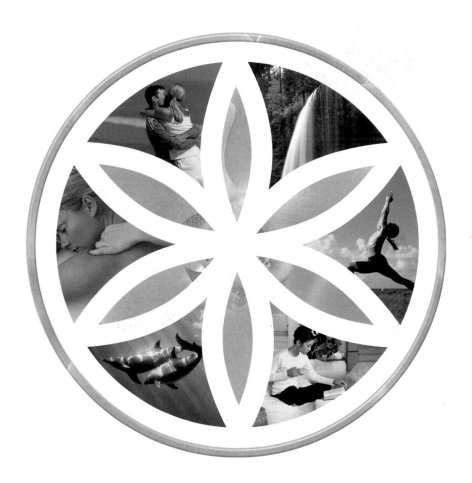

GAIAM®